COLOR GUIDE

Infectious Diseases

A.P. Ball FRCPEd

Infectious Diseases Unit
Cameron Hospital
Windygates
Fife
Scotland

J.A. Gray FRCPEd

Regional Infectious Diseases Unit
City Hospital
Edinburgh
Scotland

Churchill Livingstone

EDINBURGH LONDON MADRID MELBOURNE NEW YORK AND TOKYO 1993

CHURCHILL LIVINGSTONE
Medical Division of Longman Group UK Limited

Distributed in the United States of America by
Churchill Livingstone Inc., 650 Avenue of the Americas,
New York, N.Y. 10011, and by associated companies,
branches and representatives throughout the world.

© Longman Group UK Limited 1993

First published as Colour Aids—Infectious Diseases 1984
First published as Colour Guide—Infectious Diseases 1992
First published as Color Guide—Infectious Diseases 1993

ISBN 0-443-05093-7

British Library Cataloguing in Publication Data
A catalogue record for this book is available from the British
Library.

Library of Congress Cataloguing in Publication Data
A catalogue record for this book is available from the Library
of Congress.

Produced by Longman Group (F.E.) Ltd
Printed in Hong Kong

Acknowledgements

The authors gratefully acknowledge the kind permission of the following colleagues and others to reproduce photographs from their collections: Dr E. Edmond (Fig. 12), Dr R. Hume (Figs 33, 55, 56), Dr B. Dhillon (Figs 57, 152), Dr P. Buxton (Figs 37, 38), Dr D. Kennedy (Fig. 39), Dr P. Welsby (Fig. 40), Dr M. McDonald (Figs 53, 54), Dr B. Watt (Fig. 63), Dr A. Scott (Fig. 94), Dr J. Innes (Fig. 120), Dr D. Felix (Figs 149, 150, 151) and Abbott Laboratories Ltd (Figs 78, 79).

Special thanks are due to the Medical Photography Department, Victoria Hospital, Kirkcaldy, Fife.

Contents

1 / Measles

Etiology Measles virus, a single serotype paramyxovirus.

Incidence Common in pre-school and junior schoolchildren, notably in the last few months of the year. The pattern is usually sporadic or sub-epidemic but explosive outbreaks can occur if measles virus is introduced to previously unexposed communities.

Pathogenesis Case-to-case spread follows airborne droplet transmission from the respiratory tract of patients with active measles. There is no other reservoir of infection. Invasion of the upper respiratory tract and conjunctivae is followed by multiplication in lymphoid tissues and viremia. Histological appearances are characterized by a mononuclear reaction with giant cells and endothelial proliferation. Lesions are present in skin (rash), mucous membranes (Koplik's spots), lungs, gut and lymphoid tissue.

Clinical features The incubation period of about 10 d is followed by an upper respiratory catarrhal prodromal phase, with Koplik's spots on the buccal mucosa (Fig. 1) accompanied by conjunctivitis, otitis media and rhinitis (Fig. 2). The child is ill and miserable (in contrast with rubella). This is followed 24–48 h later by a dusky red maculopapular rash, commencing on the face and spreading peripherally via the trunk (Fig. 3 and Figs 4 & 5, p. 4). Uncomplicated measles lasts for 7–10 d. The rash fades leaving staining—brown macules with fine desquamation—which can persist for up to 3 wk (Fig. 6, p. 4).

Complications
- *Secondary bacterial otitis media, bronchopneumonia and purulent conjunctivitis*—usually caused by pneumococci and *Haemophilus influenzae*, but also by *Staphylococcus aureus*.
- *Obstructive laryngitis and dysentery*—both associated with childhood and infant malnutrition in developing countries.

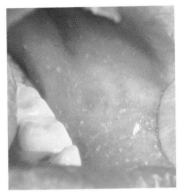

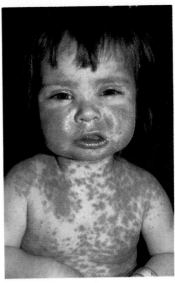

Fig. 1 Koplik's spots on buccal mucosa.

Fig. 2 Morbilliform rash, conjunctivitis and rhinitis.

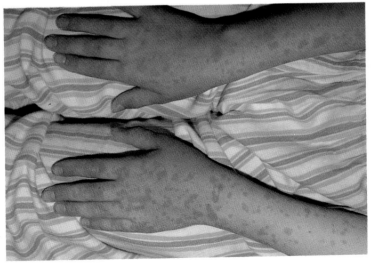

Fig. 3 Detail of measles rash.

Complications *(contd)*	• *Appendicitis*—increased incidence in measles. • *Giant cell pneumonitis*—a rare diffuse pulmonary infiltration causing respiratory failure. • *Allergic encephalomyelitis*—onset 1–2 wk after measles. Incidence 1:6000 cases. • *Sub-acute sclerosing panencephalitis*—reactivation of latent virus within brain after 5–7 yr causing fatal encephalitis. Death is inevitable within 6–12 mth. Incidence 1:1 000 000 cases. • *Atypical measles*—hyperpyrexia, vesicular rash and pneumonia. Usually seen in adults who received inactivated vaccine in the 1960s.
Treatment	Management is largely symptomatic. Erythromycin (30 mg/kg/d) or amoxicillin–clavulanic acid combination is effective for bacterial complications. There is no effective antiviral therapy for acute complications such as pneumonitis. Steroids are of marginal value in allergic encephalitis.
Prevention	Notifiable: hospitalized cases must be isolated. • *Active immunization*—live attenuated vaccine gives 97% seroconversion and long term immunity. About 3% of vaccinees develop a mild febrile reaction. Immunization is accomplished using combined measles/mumps/rubella (MMR) vaccine given between 12–18 months of age. • *Passive immunization*—human normal immunoglobulin protects if given within 72 h of exposure. This is useful in immunocompromised non-immune children.

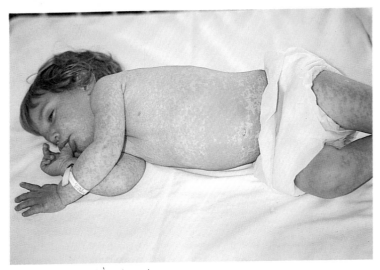

Fig. 4 Fully developed measles rash.

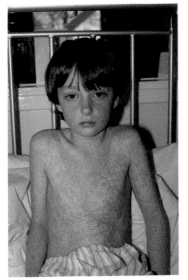

Fig. 5 Fully developed measles rash.

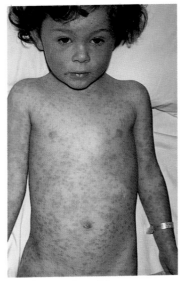

Fig. 6 Post-measles staining.

2 / Rubella

Etiology
: Rubella virus, a single serotype togavirus.

Incidence
: Common in schoolchildren with occasional epidemic fluctuations.

Pathogenesis
: Case-to-case airborne droplet transmission from the respiratory tract of active cases. Invasion by the upper respiratory tract is followed by dissemination to skin, conjunctivae and mucous membranes and a resultant mild mononuclear reaction and proliferative hyperplasia in lymph nodes. Lesions occur in the skin, lymphoid tissue, conjunctivae.

Clinical features
: The incubation period of $2\frac{1}{2}$–3 wk is followed by mild upper respiratory catarrh, conjunctival suffusion and, within 24–48 h, a discrete maculopapular generalized rash (Figs 7–10). Lymphadenopathy is prominent, notably of suboccipital and postauricular groups. Systemic upset and irritability are minimal. The rash may last 5 d but is often fleeting and fades without staining or desquamation. Rubella is diagnosed by the hemagglutination-inhibition and IgM tests.

Complications
: • *Immune complex arthritis*—typically affecting small joints, develops in 10% of women.
  • *Allergic encephalomyelitis*—commences 10–14 d after rubella. Incidence 1:6000.
  • *Purpura*—caused by thrombocytopenia and vascular defects (rare).
  • *Congenital rubella syndrome*—(p. 7).

Treatment
: Management is symptomatic. Non-steroidal anti-inflammatory agents may be required for rubella arthritis.

Prevention
: Notifiable: hospitalized cases must be isolated. Live attenuated rubella vaccines (Cendehill and RA27/3 strains) give high level protection. Immunization is accomplished using combined measles/mumps/rubella (MMR) vaccine given between 12–18 months of age.

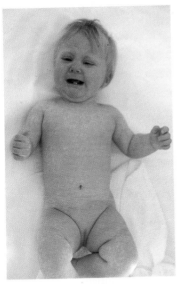

Fig. 7 Infantile rubella rash.

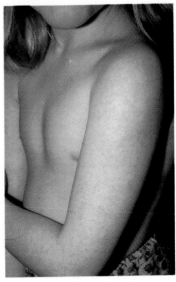

Fig. 8 Discrete pink macular rash.

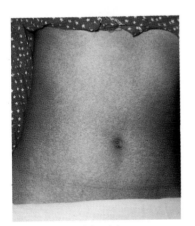

Fig. 9 Profuse rash in adult.

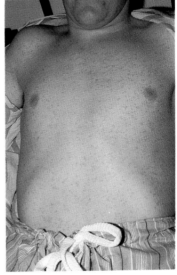

Fig. 10 Sparse rubella rash in adult.

3 / Congenital rubella syndrome (CRS)

Etiology Rubella virus (p. 5).

Incidence Affects up to 40% of fetuses exposed to maternal rubella during first trimester. Less than 10 cases per year are reported in the US.

Pathogenesis Follows transplacental fetal infection by rubella virus. Highest risk between 6–8 wk gestation, but possible risk up to 16–18 wk. Widespread fetal involvement includes persistent infection of liver, heart, CNS, lungs, pancreas and long bones. Neonatal jaundice and purpura are often present. Dysorganogenesis results in major ophthalmic, cardiac, auditory and neurological abnormalities in 10% of affected pregnancies.

Clinical features Severe CRS may include: pulmonary stenosis, patent ductus arteriosus (common), coarctation and ventricular septal defect (rare) (Fig. 11); microphthalmia, cataract (Fig. 12) and retinitis; sensorineural deafness and microcephaly. Severe mental deficiency is uncommon. The extended syndrome may include purpura, anemia, metaphyseal dysplasia, hepatitis, myocarditis, pneumonitis and low birth weight.

Treatment Non-immune mothers who develop clinical or serological evidence of rubella in early pregnancy (<15 wk) are offered therapeutic abortion. Rubella immune globulin does not prevent congenital rubella.

Prevention Immunization is accomplished using combined measles/mumps/rubella (MMR) vaccine given between 12–18 months of age. Non-immune pregnant women exposed to rubella who do not seroconvert must be immunized in the immediate puerperium. The live attenuated (RA27/3 strain) vaccines available for this purpose, must never be administered during pregnancy.

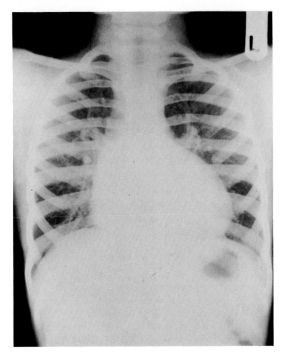

Fig. 11 Congenital ventricular septal defect.

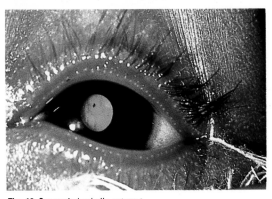

Fig. 12 Congenital rubella cataract.

4 / Mumps

Etiology	Mumps virus, a single serotype paramyxovirus.
Incidence	All ages may be affected; more common in children over 1 yr. Subclinical infection is common. Worldwide distribution. Four-year cycles, clustering in spring and winter.
Pathogenesis	Moderately infectious: spreads by airborne droplet transmission from active cases. This is followed by viremia and glandular involvement. Salivary glands—interstitial edema and lymphocyte invasion. Testes—edema, perivascular lymphocyte invasion, focal hemorrhage, destruction of germinal epithelium and tubular plugging. The CNS, pancreas, ovaries, breasts, thyroid and joints are less frequently involved.
Clinical features	The incubation period of 14–18 d is followed by a generalized febrile illness, sometimes associated with convulsions in small children. Tender parotid or submandibular gland swelling (Figs 13 & 14), bilateral in 70%, surrounded by edema, lasts for a few days. Meningeal irritation is common. Mumps virus is easily cultured from saliva or CSF. Paired sera show an antibody titre rise.
Complications	• *Orchitis* in 20% of postpubertal males (Fig. 15). *Bilateral orchitis* may result in subfertility. • *Lymphocytic meningitis* (frequent). • Post-infectious *encephalitis, pancreatitis, oophoritis* and *thyroiditis* are all rare. *Arthritis* of larger joints infrequently occurs.
Treatment	Symptomatic. Prednisone may relieve orchitis.
Prevention	Notifiable. A live attenuated mumps vaccine is available for childhood immunization: mumps meningitis may rarely follow after 3 wk. Immunization is accomplished using combined measles/mumps/rubella (MMR) vaccine given between 12–18 mth of age.

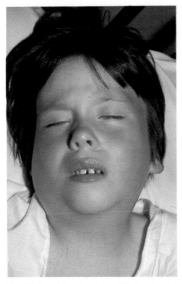

Fig. 13 Parotid and submandibular gland swelling.

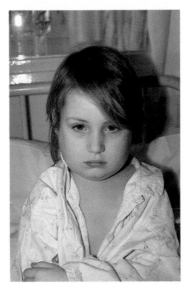

Fig. 14 Mumps parotitis.

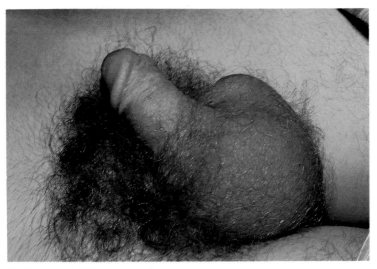

Fig. 15 Mumps orchitis.

5 / Chickenpox

Etiology Varicella-zoster virus: a DNA-containing herpes virus. Synonyms: varicella, herpes zoster.

Incidence Worldwide distribution: common in children after 9 mth, with clusters in winter and early spring. Less common but more severe in adults. Congenital and neonatal chickenpox are rare.

Pathogenesis Highly infectious: spreads by airborne droplet transmission from active cases of chickenpox (and shingles). Histologically identical skin lesions occur in the middle and deep epidermis in both chickenpox and shingles. Cell damage produces edema which forms clear vesicle fluid. This transforms into a cloudy pustule after WBC invade and then a scab which separates leaving a fine papery scar. The base of the lesion contains intranuclear inclusions and multinucleate giant cells. An enanthem (mucosal rash) is common. Chickenpox may rarely cause a hemorrhagic, edematous, necrotic pneumonia which is more common and severe in immunocompromised patients. Miliary calcification may follow. Encephalitis is unusual.

Keratitis and corneal ulcers are seen less often than with herpes simplex infections. Hemorrhagic chickenpox results from thrombocytopenia and consumption coagulopathy.

Clinical features The incubation period is about 2 wk (range 7–23 d). Influenza-like symptoms may precede the rash in adults but in children the rash (Figs 16 & 17) starts first, often with little fever. Each spot starts as a macule then progresses through vesicular, pustular and crusting stages unless aborted by antiviral agents. Crops of spots occur every day or two (Fig. 18). The scalp, face, trunk and hollows of the body are more affected than the limbs and prominences. The rash is accompanied by an enanthem (Figs 16 & 19) and may be very sparse or, notably in immunocompromised patients, profuse (Fig. 20, p. 14).

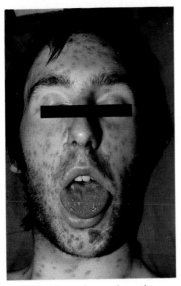

Fig. 16 Facial exanthem and enanthem on tongue.

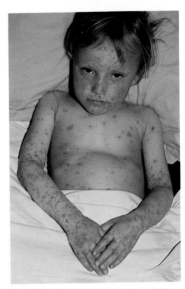

Fig. 17 Distribution in eczematous child (atypical).

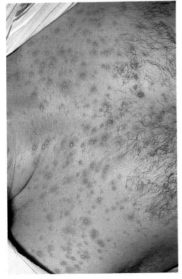

Fig. 18 Crops of papules, vesicles and pustules.

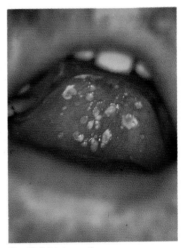

Fig. 19 Palatal enanthem.

Clinical features
(contd)

The uncomplicated illness lasts about 7 d.
Diagnosis is confirmed by virus isolation from vesicle fluid and rising antibody titres.

Complications

Secondary bacterial infection of the spots causes septic lesions or progresses to *varicella gangrenosa* (Fig. 21). Neonates, the elderly or immunodeficient patients may develop severe *pneumonia* (Figs 22 & 23). A rare and usually transient *encephalopathy*, predominantly affecting the cerebellum and characterized by ataxia and nystagmus (more rarely causing altered consciousness), can complicate chickenpox.

After primary chickenpox, varicella-zoster virus persists for life in neurological tissue. Reactivation from such foci is the cause of *herpes zoster* (shingles, p. 15) which may occur in 30% or more of patients aged >60 yrs.

Treatment

Management is largely symptomatic. Secondary skin sepsis, usually caused by staphylococci or streptococci, may require oral erythromycin. Alternative therapy is with one of the cephalosporins. Intravenous (or high dose oral—800 mg, 5 times daily in adults) acyclovir, a nucleoside antiviral agent, is highly effective in severely ill neonates or the immunosuppressed but is not used for routine childhood infections. It does not eradicate neurologically-sequestered, non-replicating virus and therefore does not prevent later zoster (shingles).

Prevention

Notifiable. Patients should be isolated from non-immune or immunocompromised patients. Zoster immune globulin may prevent disease in vulnerable contacts. Vaccines are in development.

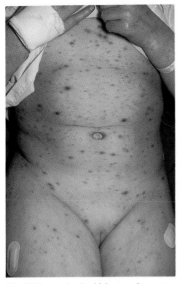

Fig. 20 Hemorrhagic chickenpox in acute leukemia.

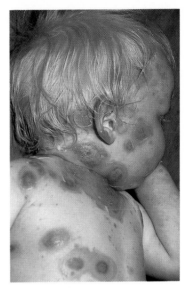

Fig. 21 Varicella gangrenosa.

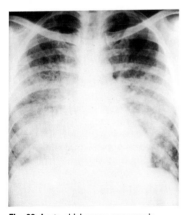

Fig. 22 Acute chickenpox pneumonia.

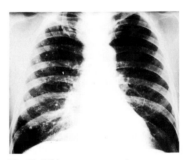

Fig. 23 Chickenpox pneumonia: late calcification.

6 / Herpes zoster (shingles)

Etiology The varicella-zoster (V–Z) virus: a DNA-containing herpes virus.

Incidence Worldwide distribution (as chickenpox) but no seasonal variation. Common in the elderly (30% incidence in those aged >60 yr), rare in childhood.

Pathogenesis Skin lesions in herpes zoster are histologically identical to chickenpox but follow sensory cranial or peripheral nerve root distributions with inflammation and necrosis of ganglion cells. Motor cells are infrequently affected. Widespread lesions occur in the immunocompromised. V–Z virus is neurotropic, often lying dormant in CNS tissue for many years after childhood chickenpox, until reactivated. Reactivation can complicate immunosuppression due to malignancy, corticosteroid and cytotoxic drugs or radiotherapy but such precipitants are usually absent. Shingles is less infectious than chickenpox.

Clinical features Burning pain or paraesthesia in the affected dermatome are the usual presenting features. Pain can be mild or severe and of short or long duration, sometimes being replaced by protracted post-herpetic neuralgia. A day or so after the pain starts, skin lesions appear, confined to the affected dermatome with evolution from macule, through vesicle, pustule, crust and scar as in chickenpox. Vesiculopustular lesions often coalesce. A girdle-like eruption following a unilateral thoracic dermatome is the most common manifestation (Figs 24 & 25, and Fig. 29, p. 18), but any sensory nerve can be affected, e.g. supraclavicular nerves (Fig. 28, p. 18). Sacral shingles may interfere with bladder and bowel function. Limb girdle or peripheral limb involvement may be associated with mixed motor and sensory disturbance.

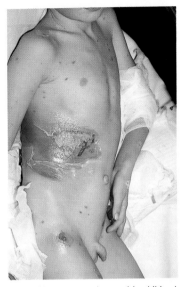

Fig. 24 Herpes zoster (unusual in children).

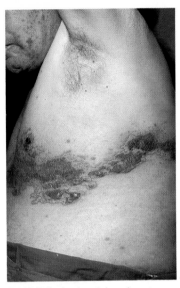

Fig. 25 Fully developed thoracic zoster: limited to single dermatome.

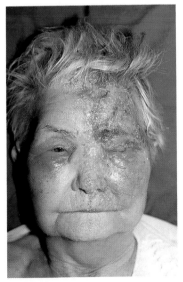

Fig. 26 Early ophthalmic zoster with secondary infection.

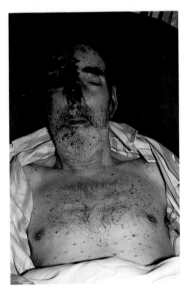

Fig. 27 Late ophthalmic zoster: generalized rash in leukemia.

Clinical features
(contd)

Motor and sensory involvement is typical of the Ramsay–Hunt syndrome (Fig. 30) comprising ear pain, vesicles on the external auditory meatus, with facial palsy and loss of taste. Any branch of the trigeminal nerve may be affected, but herpes zoster ophthalmicus is commonest (Figs 26 & 27, p. 16). When the nasociliary branch is involved, corneal damage may result. Virus may be grown on tissue culture from the skin lesions. Antibody titres rise during the illness in most patients.

Complications

Secondary bacterial infection may occur. In immunocompromised patients *extensive disseminated skin lesions* resemble chickenpox. *Pneumonia* and *meningoencephalitis* are uncommon. *Post-herpetic neuralgia*, a common sequel within affected dermatome(s), produces transient but severe attacks of pain, persisting for months.

Treatment

Analgesics are usually required. Secondary staphylococcal or streptococcal infection responds to oral erythromycin. Alternative therapy is with one of the cephalosporins. Oral acyclovir (800 mg 5 times daily) for 7–10 d given early can arrest progression and is especially useful for ophthalmic, sacral and motor disease. Severe generalized chickenpox complicating zoster in elderly or immunocompromised patients may require i.v. acyclovir. Ophthalmic zoster with conjunctival involvement requires topical chloramphenicol, acyclovir and corticosteroids. Post-herpetic neuralgia may respond to carbamazepine, transcutaneous nerve stimulation or nerve obliteration.

Prevention

Once acquired, V–Z virus may erupt as shingles at any time. This is not preventable. Patients with zoster are infectious and should be isolated.

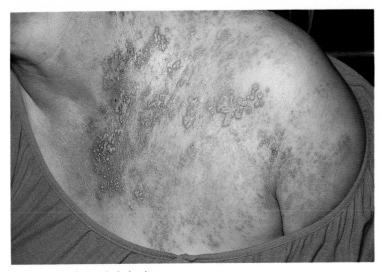

Fig. 28 Zoster of supraclavicular dermatomes.

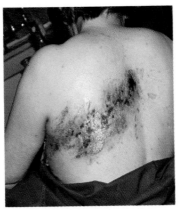

Fig. 29 Healing of thoracic zoster.

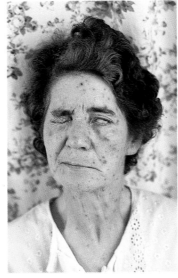

Fig. 30 Ramsay–Hunt syndrome: facial palsy.

7 / Herpes simplex infections

Etiology	Two DNA-containing viruses, distinguishable epidemiologically, clinically and serologically as herpes simplex types 1 and 2 (HSV-1 and HSV-2). Synonyms: *Herpesvirus hominis* I/II.
Incidence	Primary HSV-1 infection is usually acquired in infancy by the airborne droplet route. Congenital infection with HSV-1 is rare. Congenital HSV-2 disease may occur but is less common than perinatal infection acquired from the maternal birth canal. Most HSV-2 infection in adults is sexually acquired especially by homosexuals and the promiscuous.
Pathogenesis	Non-immunes are vulnerable to virus shed from the skin and mucosa of active cases over several days. HSV-1 usually affects the mucocutaneous junctions of lips and nose and HSV-2 the genitalia. Virus replication in the epithelium or mucosa causes inflammation, cell lysis and thin walled vesicles. After primary infection HSV-1 and HSV-2 migrate to nerves where they lie dormant. Reactivation may be precipitated by bacterial infection (herpes febrilis), sunlight, menstruation and immunosuppression.
Clinical features	Primary HSV-1 stomatitis consists of painful ulcerating vesicles on the lips, anterior buccal mucosa and nares (Figs 31 & 32). Dendritic corneal ulcers can cause blindness and are more common in HSV-1 than HSV-2 infections. Congenital HSV-1 or HSV-2 infection (Fig. 33) causes jaundice, thombocytopenia, hepatosplenomegaly, rashes, encephalopathy and choroidoretinitis. In eczematous patients HSV-1 infection may be widespread (Kaposi's varicelliform eruption, eczema herpeticum (Fig. 34, p. 22). Similar eruptions may be the presenting features of AIDS (p. 109) or of other diseases associated with immunosuppression, e.g. lymphoma.

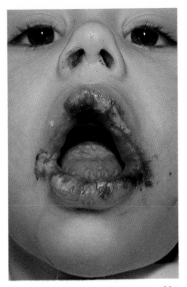

Fig. 31 Primary herpes simplex stomatitis.

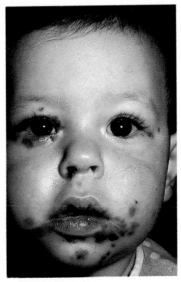

Fig. 32 Primary stomatitis with skin, nasal and periocular involvement.

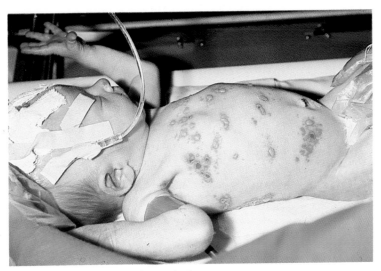

Fig. 33 Congenital disseminated herpes simplex.

Clinical features
(contd)

Primary HSV-2 infection usually affects the genitalia or anus with clusters of painful vesicles lasting for 10 d (Fig. 36). Health care workers may be infected on the fingers, resulting in herpetic whitlow (Fig. 35). HSV-1 encephalitis may complicate neonatal, primary or asymptomatic reactivation of virus with focal CNS signs, confusion and coma. CSF is often normal and culture-negative but CT brain scanning shows focal disease.

Virus can be isolated from the infected mouth, anus and genitalia and, in encephalitis, from brain biopsy but usually not from CSF. Serology is diagnostic in primary infections but is of little value during reactivations or encephalitis.

Treatment

Most routine HSV-1 infections are localized and require no specific therapy. Corneal ulceration should be treated with acyclovir (steroids are contraindicated). Secondary infection by oral anaerobes in stomatitis may benefit from metronidazole or penicillin V.

The period of discomfort and virus shedding from acute HSV-2 lesions is reduced by oral acyclovir. Single courses of acyclovir do not prevent subsequent recurrences but extended therapy (for 3 mth) can reduce their frequency in patients with regular attacks. Intravenous acyclovir is the treatment of choice in encephalitis and disseminated infection, significantly reducing mortality and residual neurological damage.

Prevention

Active cases should be isolated from babies and the immunosuppressed. Health care personnel with herpetic whitlows or other active lesions should not work with infants or the immunosuppressed. Sexual activity should be avoided in acute HSV-2 disease. Experimental vaccines are under evaluation.

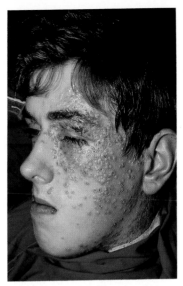

Fig. 34 Kaposi's varicelliform eruption (eczema herpeticum).

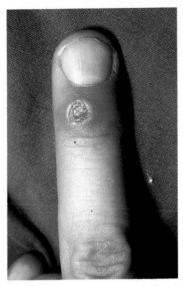

Fig. 35 Herpetic whitlow (surgeon's finger).

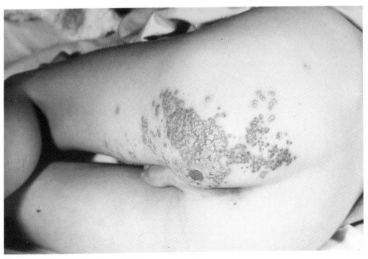

Fig. 36 Herpes simplex type 2 (child, non-venereal).

8 / Erythema infectiosum (slapped cheek disease)

Etiology The human parvovirus B19 (HPV B19).

Incidence Worldwide distribution, most common in children aged 4–15 yr.

Pathogenesis Spread occurs via respiratory droplet emission from active cases. Up to 30% of household contacts are affected. HPV B19 multiplies in rapidly dividing cells, notably red cell precursors (which may lyse). Viremia follows in 5–7 d. Rash and arthritis result from a host–virus interaction, probably immune-complex mediated. Aplastic crises and hemolytic anemias may follow erythroid dysplasia. A third of intrauterine HPV B19 infections cause hydrops fetalis or stillbirths.

Clinical features **Erythema infectiosum:** the incubation period (5–10 d) is followed by non-tender erythema of the cheeks (Fig. 37), followed by the characteristic lace-like rash over the limbs and trunk (Fig. 38). The rash is more common in older children. These features persist for 7–10 d.

Arthritis: most common in adult contacts, usually producing symmetrical arthralgia lasting several wk.

Aplastic crises: HPV B19 is the most common cause of aplastic crises in patients with sickle cell anemia and also causes aplasia in patients with other forms of chronic hemolytic anemia.

Immunodeficient patients: chronic infection may cause severe persistent anemia or transient aplasia.

Serology for specific IgM and IgG antibodies is available but culture for HPV B19 is not normally undertaken.

Treatment and prevention Treatment is symptomatic: arthritis responds to NSAIDs. Vaccines have not been developed.

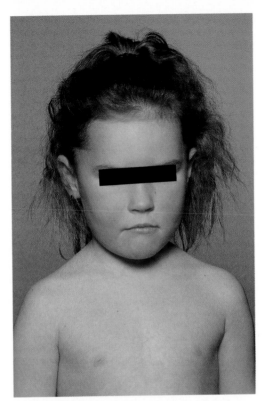

Fig. 37 Facial (slapped cheek) appearance.

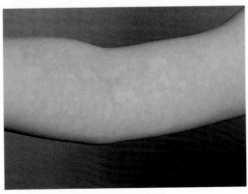

Fig. 38 Typical lace-like skin rash (adult).

9 / Kawasaki (mucocutaneous lymph node) syndrome

Etiology Unknown: presumed transmissable on epidemiological grounds.

Incidence Worldwide, affecting children, particularly asiatics and blacks. Mini-epidemics in winter/spring based on background endemicity.

Pathogenesis Presumed to be an immunological reaction to an infectious agent. Immune complexes and activated B cells (producing IgG/IgM) circulate, resulting in inflammatory vasculitis, resembling infant polyarteritis and affecting joints and coronary arteries.

Clinical features **Acute febrile phase:** lasting 7–10 d, characterized by fever of >5 d duration, conjunctivitis, fissuring of lips, mucosal injection, strawberry tongue, swelling of extremities, cervical lymphadenopathy, erythema and rashes (Fig. 39).

Sub-acute phase: lasting 2 wk thereafter with resolution of acute signs. Desquamation is prominent (Fig. 40), accompanied by arthritis and thrombocytosis. Myocardial dysfunction may appear.

Convalescent phase: acute signs disappear—the ESR remains elevated for up to 10 wk. Significant coronary artery (CA) involvement occurs in >20%.

Coronary artery disease: the prognosis is usually good but some develop aneurysm (Fig. 41), stenosis and occlusion. Mortality of 2% follows myocardial failure/infarction. Risk factors include male Caucasians, age <1 yr, prolonged fever, high IgE, arrhythmias and cardiomegaly.

Definitive serology is not available. Laboratory findings include leucocytosis, anemia, high ESR and IgE, and, typically, thrombocytosis peaking at 3 wk. Coronary arteries should be assessed by biplanar echocardiography in sub-acute and convalescent phases.

Treatment and prevention Aspirin (80 mg/kg/day) commenced on diagnosis, is reduced (3–5 mg/kg/day) in convalescence. Early i.v. immunoglobulin therapy (400 mg/kg/day) concomitant with aspirin therapy may prevent coronary artery damage. Corticosteroids are contraindicated.

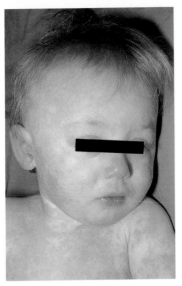

Fig. 39 Erythematous rash, conjunctivitis and sore lips.

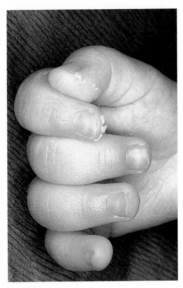

Fig. 40 Peri-ungual desquamation.

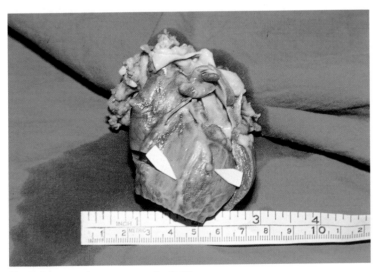

Fig. 41 Coronary artery aneurysms at autopsy.

10 / Orf

Etiology	Orf virus: an ovoid paravaccinia virus.
Incidence	A common worldwide zoonosis of sheep and goats in which it causes watery papillomatous lesions on the mucosa and conjunctivae. Man is infected by direct occupational contact with the animal, most commonly during spring lambing. Now relatively rare due to preventive veterinary vaccination.
Pathogenesis	A nodule appears at the site of contact where virus enters through a laceration or abrasion of the skin. A vesiculobulbous hyperplastic mass develops, usually without further spread.
Clinical features	Shepherds are infected at lambing time but shearers, abattoir workers and veterinary surgeons can also catch orf. Exposed surfaces such as hands, forearms or the face are usually affected. An irritating but pain-free nodule develops, enlarges and has a gelatinous appearance (Fig. 42). It may be incised (wrongly) but no material expressed. Healing (Fig. 43) takes some weeks but there is no scarring. Secondary bacterial cellulitis or lymphangitis may occur. Erythema multiforme is an occasional complication. Virus can be isolated from the lesion and demonstrated by electron microscopy.
Treatment	No specific treatment is available. Erythromycin is effective for secondary bacterial infection. Alternative therapy is with one of the cephalosporins. The lesion should not be incised.
Prevention	Gloves should be worn when handling infected animals. Isolation of patients is unnecessary. An effective ovine vaccine is now available which prevents enzootic disease in sheep.

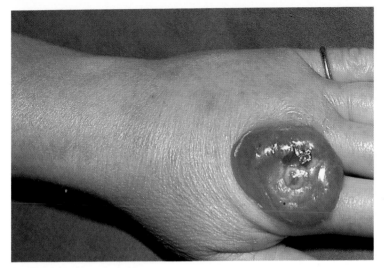

Fig. 42 Acute orf in a shepherdess.

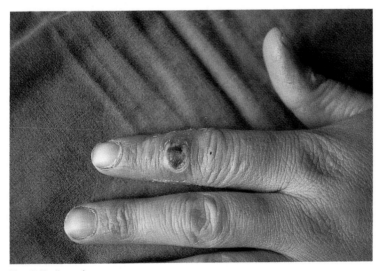

Fig. 43 Healing orf.

11 / Herpangina

Etiology   Coxsackie A viruses types 1–6, 8, 10 (commonly) and other types (rare).

Incidence   Predominantly sporadic, but subject to minor epidemic fluctuations. May be accompanied by an upsurge of viral meningitis, enteritis and infantile febrile episodes due to the same epidemic type. A significant proportion of infections are asymptomatic or trivial.

Pathogenesis   Spread occurs mainly by the fecal–oral route and, less commonly, via airborne droplet emission, usually among young schoolchildren who transmit infection to older siblings and parents.

Clinical features   Herpangina is characterized by fever, moderate systemic toxemia and ulcerative pharyngitis. The onset is acute and resolution may take up to a week. Fluctuant pyrexia is present for the initial few days accompanied by ulcers of the palatal pillars, posterior soft palate and uvula (and less commonly of the tonsils and posterior aspect of the tongue) (Fig. 44). The ulcers are 1–5 mm in size, are covered by necrotic slough, and spare the anterior of the mouth—in contrast with herpes simplex stomatitis and Stevens–Johnson syndrome. There is no accompanying rash. Complicating parotitis has been described. Diagnosis is primarily clinical but may be supported by virus isolation from throat and stool. Serology may reveal a diagnostic rise in antibody titre.

Treatment   No specific therapy is available and antibiotics are not indicated. Symptomatic relief may be obtained with aspirin gargles.

Prevention   Not notifiable: isolation not necessary. No specific preventive measures are available.

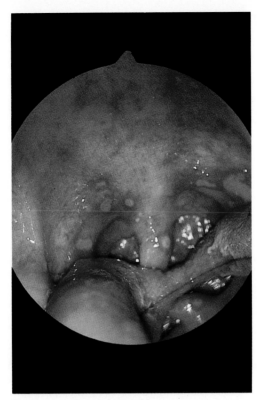

Fig. 44 Herpangina: ulceration of fauces.

12 / Hand, foot and mouth disease

Etiology   Coxsackie virus A16 (occasionally A5 or A10).

Incidence   This unusual clinical manifestation of enteroviral activity is associated with clusters of clinical cases when infection is widespread in the community. Virus is often isolated from asymptomatic family contacts. Worldwide distribution but probably more common in temperate zones.

Pathogenesis   Spreads primarily by fecal–oral transmission from active cases and convalescent excretors—probably also by the airborne droplet route from active cases. Viremia is followed by a typically distributed peripheral skin rash and accompanying oral lesions.

Clinical features   The incubation period is 3–7 d and is followed by the appearance of bright red spots or small vesicles on the buccal mucosa, which ulcerate and then heal within 7–10 d. The ulcers, which are painful, spare the back of the throat and affect mainly the lips, tongue, and inside of the cheeks and palate. A sparse, painless rash of the hands and feet affects the lateral aspects of fingers and toes but also involves the palm and soles. The skin lesions (Figs 45 & 46) vary from red macules to small vesicles, containing milky fluid, and bullae which may ulcerate and heal 7–10 d later. In infancy the buttocks may be affected. In children, mild fever and malaise are common but adults usually have little systemic upset. There are no specific complications. Virus can be isolated by tissue culture or material from oral and skin lesions. Specific serum antibodies show a diagnostic rise in titre.

Treatment   Management is symptomatic only. Antibiotics are not indicated.

Prevention   Good hygiene—although by the time of diagnosis other household members will already be infected, whether symptomatic or not.

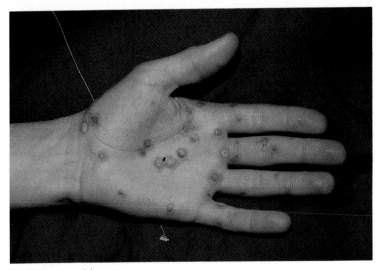

Fig. 45 Palmar vesicles.

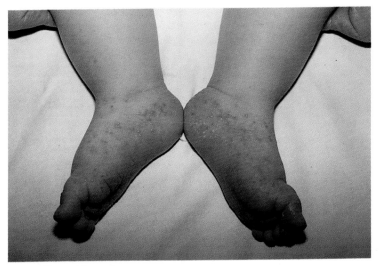

Fig. 46 Milky vesicles on feet.

13 / Infectious mononucleosis (IM)

Etiology   Epstein–Barr virus (EBV), a herpes virus. Similar illnesses may be caused by toxoplasmosis (p. 37), cytomegalovirus infection (p. 39) and primary HIV infection (p. 107).

Incidence   Worldwide distribution causing glandular fever (Europe and N. America). EBV is also associated with Burkitt's lymphoma (Africa) and nasopharyngeal carcinoma (Far East). Inapparent infection is common, especially in lower socioeconomic groups. Clinical glandular fever is most often seen among affluent adolescents.

Pathogenesis   Close contact and kissing facilitate transmission of EBV from saliva. The individual transmitting the illness is often asymptomatic. After oropharyngeal invasion, virus infects B-lymphocytes which form heterophile antibody. Some B-cells are transformed and EBV-containing B-cells continue to replicate. Next, killer T-cells destroy some EBV infected B-cells and suppressor T-cells limit B-cell transformation. The T-cell response causes the lymph node and splenic enlargement, anginose sore throat and the characteristic atypical lymphocytes seen in the peripheral blood. Later a long-lasting balance ensues between infected B-cells and killer T-cells. If transformed B-cells proliferate, in the absence of T-cells, or if virus overwhelms B-cells causing agammaglobulinemia, fulminating disease results.

Clinical features   The incubation period of about 4–8 wk is followed by an illness of 2–3 wk duration, characterized by sore throat, malaise, fever, splenomegaly and generalized tender lymphadenopathy. Pus and pseudomembrane cover the tonsils (Fig. 47) but clear in 1–2 wk. Cervical lymphadenopathy and periorbital edema are prominent (Fig. 48 and Fig. 50, p. 36), and palatal petechiae are typical (Fig. 49).

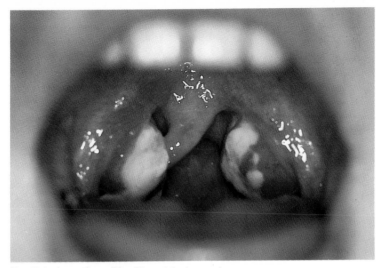

Fig. 47 Anginose pharyngitis with wash-leather exudate.

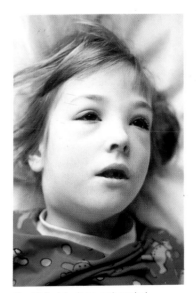

Fig. 48 Facial edema and cervical lymphadenopathy.

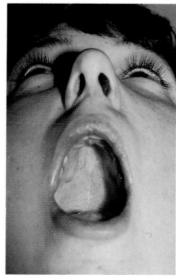

Fig. 49 Palatal petechiae.

Clinical features
(*contd*)

Hepatomegaly and mild jaundice, and a pink maculopapular rash occur less commonly (Figs 51 & 52). Life-long immunity is conferred.

A number of diagnostic investigations are available. Atypical mononuclear cells are present in the peripheral blood and the Monospot slide test and Paul Bunnell test for IgG antibodies are positive. Rising titres of EBV specific IgM and IgG antibodies can be demonstrated. Liver function tests indicate mild hepatocellular damage.

Complications

Splenic rupture, airways obstruction, blood dyscrasias or CNS complications occasionally prove fatal. *Hemolysis, thrombocytopenia, pneumonitis, encephalitis, meningitis, post-infectious polyneuropathy, lymphoma* and *myocarditis* may occur. Administration of ampicillin or amoxicillin typically causes a maculopapular skin rash in IM (Fig. 51).

Transient depression is a common sequel. Glandular fever is a frequent cause of the *post-viral fatigue syndrome* and may be associated with some cases of *myalgic encephalomyelitis.*

Treatment

Adequate rest is important. Ganciclovir therapy may globally improve symptoms but its value is not proven in routine cases. Prednisone or emergency tracheostomy are sometimes required for severe pharyngeal edema causing incipient respiratory obstruction. Superimposed streptococcal infection is treated with penicillin or erythromycin. Ampicillin or amoxicillin are contraindicated, as use will lead to a maculopapular rash in >90% of patients with mononucleosis. Complicating hemolytic anemia usually responds to prednisone and transfusion.

Prevention

No active or passive immunization is available. Strict isolation is not necessary.

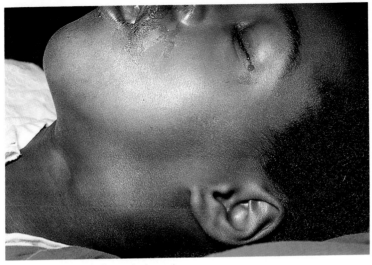

Fig. 50 Cervical lymphadenopathy (severe).

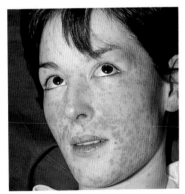

Fig. 51 Jaundice and ampicillin rash.

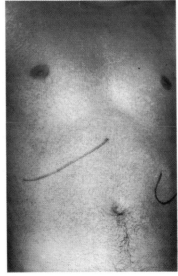

Fig. 52 Rash and hepatosplenomegaly.

14 / Toxoplasmosis

Etiology *Toxoplasma gondii*, an intracellular protozoon parasite.

Incidence Usually an asymptomatic infection, rarely producing acute disease. Congenital infection occurs in 0.1% of live births.

Pathogenesis A zoonosis, primarily a disease of cats but also of intermediates such as birds. Acquired by ingestion of oocysts, commonly from kitten feces, or by airborne droplet transmission. The parasite disseminates in reticuloendothelial and other tissues with secondary spread of trophozoites. Latent infection and transplacental fetal spread may follow.

Clinical features **Acquired disease:** mononucleosis syndrome characterized by fever, atypical mononucleosis lymphadenopathy and splenomegaly is common. Choroidoretinitis (Figs 53 & 54) and encephalitis are rare.

Congenital disease:
- *Disseminated*—jaundice, lymphadenopathy, splenomegaly and choroidoretinitis.
- *CNS disease*—hydrocephalus, convulsions, and intracranial calcification (Fig. 55). Perinatal mortality 10–20%.

Opportunistic disease: reactivation of latent infection in immunosuppressed patients may cause severe encephalitis.

Toxoplasma encephalitis: common in AIDS patients. CT scan shows focal ring-enhanced lesions.

Toxoplasmosis is diagnosed serologically (Sabin–Feldman dye test and IgM titres).

Treatment Severe ocular or CNS involvement is treated with pyrimethamine plus a sulfonamide for 3–4 wk. Clindamycin plus pyrimethamine is alternative treatment in sulfa allergic patients. Additional steroid therapy is of value in choroidoretinitis.

Prevention Isolation not necessary. No adequate control measures are available. Pregnant women should avoid kittens.

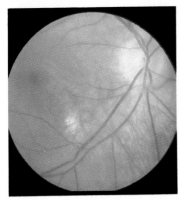

Fig. 53 Acute choroidoretinitis.

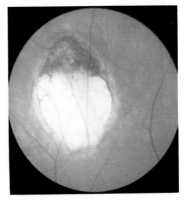

Fig. 54 Healed choroidoretinitis.

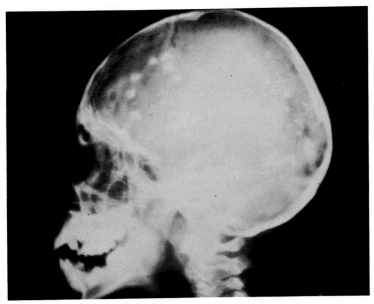

Fig. 55 Congenital intracranial calcification.

15 / Cytomegalovirus (CMV) infection

Etiology   Cytomegalovirus: a DNA-containing herpes virus.

Incidence   Worldwide distribution. Most infections are subclinical but many symptomatic intrauterine, neonatal and adult acquired infections occur. Peak incidences occur between 1 and 2 yr and 15–30 yr.

Pathogenesis   Spreads by airborne droplet transmission from infected nasopharyngeal secretions. Transplacental infection may arise from primary infection or reactivation of latent virus during pregnancy. Perinatal infection results from maternal cervical infection. Infected infants excrete virus in the urine for months. CMV-infected cells swell and show intranuclear and intracytoplasmic inclusions. Nuclear chromatin is pushed to the edge of the cell giving an 'owl's eye' appearance.

Clinical features   **Congenital CMV disease** (Fig. 56): results in choroidoretinitis, hepatosplenomegaly, jaundice, rash, microcephaly and deafness.

Acquired CMV disease: clinically indistinguishable from infectious mononucleosis although membranous pharyngitis is uncommon. Choroidoretinitis may occur. In immunosuppressed (tumor/transplant) patients primary or reactivational CMV pneumonitis has a mortality of >50%.

AIDS: CMV retinitis (Fig. 57), pneumonitis and colitis are common.

Diagnosis is established by virus isolation from tissues, urine and saliva and a rising antibody titre. An atypical lymphocytosis is usually found in peripheral blood (not in AIDS).

Treatment   Intravenous ganciclovir or foscarnet may be effective for CMV disease in AIDS/immunocompromised patients.

Prevention   Vaccine development is being undertaken. Transfusion of CMV antibody negative blood is recommended, when necessary, for immunocompromised and HIV-infected patients.

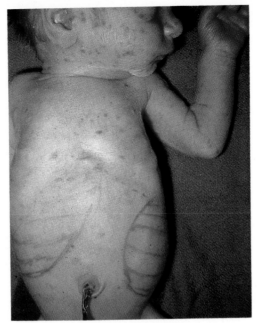

Fig. 56 Congenital rash and hepatomegaly.

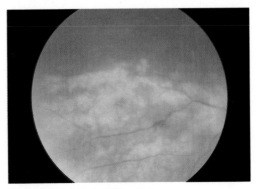

Fig. 57 CMV retinitis in AIDS patient.

16 / Viral hepatitis

Etiology   Hepatitis A (HAV), B (HBV), C (HCV), delta agent and other viruses.

Incidence   Worldwide distribution. HAV affects the young and is often subclinical. HBV accounts for over 40% of cases of acute viral hepatitis in the US. HCV is predominantly blood-transmitted.

Pathogenesis   HAV is transmitted by the fecal–oral route from active cases; HBV by contact, sexual and parenteral routes from cases and carriers; and HCV via blood products and direct contact. Neonatal HBV infection is acquired from carrier mothers. Viral hepatitis causes centrilobular hepatocyte necrosis and portal inflammation. Delta agent coinfection in HBV positive patients causes fulminant or chronic progressive hepatitis.

Clinical features   The incubation periods are: HAV 15–40 d, HBV 50–140 d, HCV 30–160 d. Illness starts with malaise, nausea, vomiting, mild fever and abdominal discomfort. Arthralgia may herald hepatitis B. A week later, after the onset of dark urine and pale stools, jaundice appears (Fig. 58). Evidence of addiction may be seen in HBV infections (Fig. 59). Altered consciousness, a flapping tremor and fetor hepaticus precede complicating coma (Fig. 60). Diagnosis is confirmed by an HAV-specific IgM response, demonstration of HBV surface antigen (Fig. 61) or by ELISA (HCV). Infections with HBV and HCV can progress to chronic hepatitis.

Treatment   Largely symptomatic. Interferon-α-2b is useful in chronic disease.

Prevention   Notification, isolation, screening of blood donors for HB_sAg and active HBV immunization. Hyperimmune anti-HBV immunoglobulin for postexposure prophylaxis, neonates of HB_sAg carrier mothers and human normal immunoglobulin for travellers to HAV areas. Active immunization against HAV infection has recently become available.

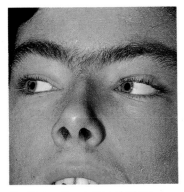

Fig. 58 Jaundice of skin and sclerae.

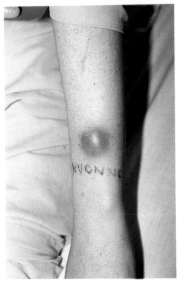

Fig. 59 Addict's arm: tattoo, needle track and abscess.

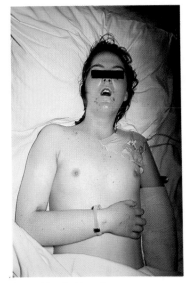

Fig. 60 Terminal hepatic coma: note bruising.

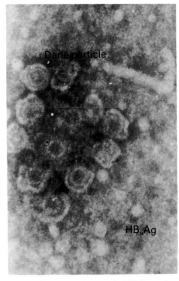

Fig. 61 Electron micrograph: HB_sAg and Dane particles (whole virus) in serum.

17 / Leptospirosis

Etiology	*Leptospira icterohaemorrhagiae, L. hebdomadis, L. canicola* etc.: pathogenic spirochetes.
Incidence	In the US, about 50 to 100 cases are reported each year; similar order of frequency in Europe but more common in tropics. Occupational risks related to rat infested environments.
Pathogenesis	Zoonosis transmitted from reservoirs in rats (*L. icterohaemorrhagiae*), cattle (*L. hebdomadis*) and dogs or pigs (*L. canicola*), usually by skin contact with urine or infected animals. Produces multisystem disease including hepatitis, nephritis, meningitis, coagulopathies and immune-complex disease.
Clinical features	**Weil's disease (L. icterohaemorrhagiae):** prodromal headache, myalgia, pyrexia, rigors and prostration, followed 1 wk later by hepatitis and nephritis, and hemorrhage caused by disseminated intravascular coagulation. Hemorrhagic herpes labialis and subconjunctival hemorrhages are often present (Fig. 62). Agglutination tests, urine cultures and dark-ground examination (Fig. 63) are usually diagnostic. **L. hebdomadis infection:** milder form of Weil's disease, often with lymphocytic meningitis. **Canicola fever (L. canicola):** prodromal syndrome less severe than Weil's disease, followed by lymphocytic meningitis.
Complications	Hepatorenal failure causes death in 10% of patients with Weil's disease. Transverse myelitis, uveitis and myopericarditis may occur.
Treatment	Penicillin G or tetracycline/doxycycline are most effective when given in the prodromal phase.
Prevention	Notification: isolation not necessary. Veterinary vaccines. Hygiene in farms, abattoirs and kennels. Tetracycline prophylaxis for hospital staff exposed to blood or urine.

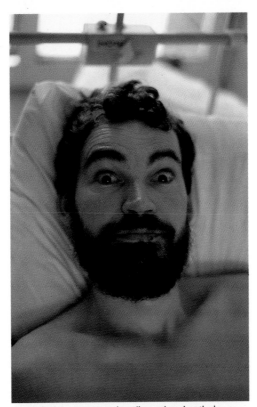

Fig. 62 Facial appearance: jaundice, subconjunctival hemorrhage, hemorrhagic herpes labialis in Weil's disease.

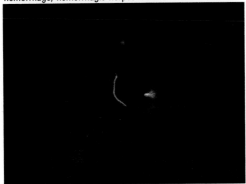

Fig. 63 Leptospirae (dark-ground examination of urine).

18 / Staphylococcal infection

Etiology	Coagulase-positive *Staphylococcus aureus*. The skin commensal *Staph. epidermidis* may infect prostheses and ventriculoatrial shunts, and is also associated with urinary tract infection in sexually active young women.
Incidence	Worldwide. Opportunistic infections occur in immunocompromised patients and diabetics.
Pathogenesis	Pathogenic staphylococci are carried on skin or anterior nares and may cause endogenous or exogenous infection by invasion, toxin production or both. Staphylococci enter skin breaches or hair follicles causing local sepsis, polymorphonuclear leucocytosis and pus formation. Invasion of bronchial mucosa devitalized by influenza leads to staphylococcal pneumonia. Superficial skin infections may result in bacteremia with endocarditis and widespread sepsis. Toxin production or absorption of preformed toxin can cause enterotoxin food poisoning, tampon-associated staphylococcal toxic shock syndrome and exfoliatin induced toxic epidermal necrolysis (TEN).
Clinical features	***Skin infections.*** Impetigo (Fig. 64) affects only the superficial epidermis and is highly infectious. A boil (Fig. 65) is an inflamed infected hair follicle from which pus may discharge spontaneously. Coalescence of infected follicles may result in a carbuncle. In cellulitis (Fig. 66) deeper tissues are infected.
	Bacteremia results from superficial or deep sepsis or from direct injection of staphylococci by drug addicts. Endocarditis may follow with widespread septic emboli to brain, lungs, skin (Fig. 67) and kidneys. Staphylococcal pneumonia commonly results in empyema and lung abscesses, notably in cystic fibrosis.

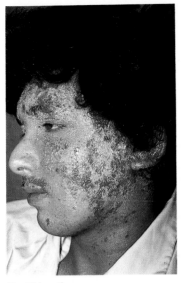

Fig. 64 Impetigo.

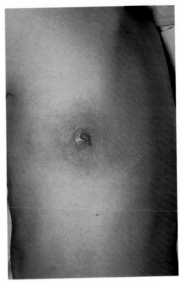

Fig. 65 Boil exuding yellow pus.

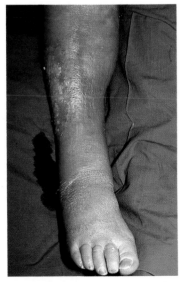

Fig. 66 Cellulitis with epidermal necrosis.

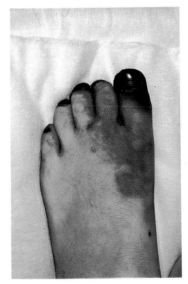

Fig. 67 Septic embolic gangrene in endocarditis.

Clinical features
(contd)

Toxin-induced disease. Staphylococcal food poisoning starts 1–2 h after eating preformed enterotoxin with profuse vomiting and prostration but without diarrhea. Exotoxin-F induced toxic or tampon shock is characterized by fever, hypotension and rash. Staphylococci are found high in the vagina but rarely in blood cultures. In TEN, infants with scalded skin syndrome (Ritter's disease: Figs 68 & 69) or children with Lyell's syndrome (Fig. 70) develop painful erythematous shearing of superficial epidermal bullae. TEN also occurs in immunocompromised adults (Fig. 71). Staphylococci can usually be isolated from affected sites except in TEN and food poisoning.

Treatment

Superficial skin sepsis is treated with dressings, poulticing or surgical drainage. Deeper or systemic infection requires urgent parenteral chemotherapy usually with oxacillin/nafcillin, vancomycin and imipenem. Alternatives are clindamycin or one of the cephalosporins. Intravenous fluids, oxygen, physiotherapy and surgical drainage of septic arthritis, lung abscess and empyema may be necessary. Prosthetic valve replacement is frequently required in endocarditis. Methicillin-resistant *Staph. aureus* (MRSA) or *Staph. epidermidis* (MRSE) infections may occur in hospital outbreaks. Treatment may require the use of vancomycin or teicoplanin with gentamicin or rifampin (consult infectious disease physicians).

Prevention

Scrupulous hand washing using alcohol-based disinfectants; asepsis in surgery and in the care of neonates; cleansing of traumatic wounds; isolation and/or treatment of staphylococcal carriers; improved food hygiene; use of gloves.

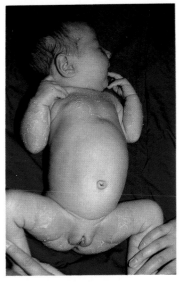

Fig. 68 Ritter's disease.

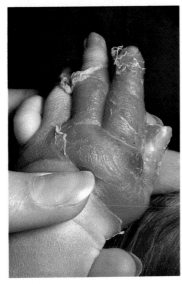

Fig. 69 Ritter's disease.

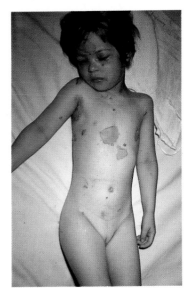

Fig. 70 Lyell's syndrome.

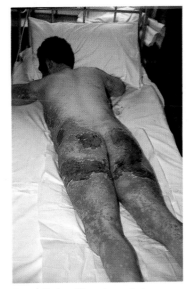

Fig. 71 Toxic epidermal necrolysis (lymphoma patient).

19 / Osteomyelitis (OM)

Etiology   *Staphylococcus aureus* causes 80% of cases of OM, most of the remainder being due to *Strep. pyogenes, H. influenzae* and, less commonly, enterobacteria.

Incidence   Staphylococcal OM is most common in males aged between 3 and 10 yr. Distribution is worldwide but more common in warm climates and among those with sickle cell disease and diabetes mellitus. Prosthetic hip joints may become infected.

Pathogenesis   During bacteremia, which is often asymptomatic or trivial, staphylococci settle in metaphyses or sites of bone injury. About 60–70% of staphylococcal OM occurs in the easily traumatized lower limbs. Local inflammation leads to pus formation, periosteal elevation and bone necrosis secondary to septic thrombosis.

Clinical features   A history of injury may be given. The onset is sudden with fever, rigors and exquisitely tender local inflammation in the bone or joint. Untreated, septic sinus formation (Fig. 72), bone necrosis leading to sequestrum formation (Fig. 73) and pathological fracture occur. The causal organism can be identified in blood (50–60% positive), bone biopsy and joint fluid cultures. Leucocytosis is usual. X-ray changes take several weeks to develop. Isotope bone scanning may assist but should not delay onset of treatment.

Treatment   Antibiotics are given for 6 wk. Nafcillin/oxacillin or, alternatively, clindamycin or an antistaphylococcal cephalosporin give good results in staphylococcal OM. Chronic disease may require 1–2 yrs treatment. Oral ciprofloxacin or i.v. cephalosporins (e.g. ceftriaxone, ceftazidime) and aminoglycosides are useful for Gram-negative and pseudomonal OM. Other organisms are treated according to their sensitivities. Surgical drainage and/or sequestrectomy are required in 50%.

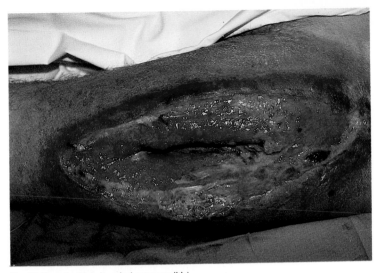

Fig. 72 Sinus in thigh (surgical osteomyelitis).

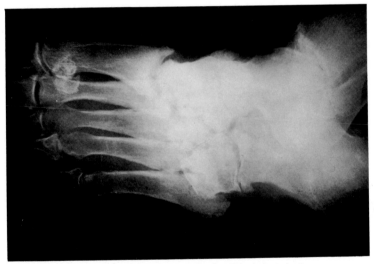

Fig. 73 Disorganized tarsus (osteomyelitis complicating diabetic foot ulcer).

20 / Infections with *Streptococcus pyogenes*

Etiology — Beta-hemolytic streptococci: classified by cell wall carbohydrates into Lancefield's groups and by T-proteins into Griffith's types.

Incidence — Worldwide distribution. Pyoderma mainly affects children with poor hygiene in the tropics. Scarlet fever, rheumatic fever and post-streptococcal glomerulonephritis are rare except in the developing world but a resurgence of rheumatic fever is now being encountered in the US.

Pathogenesis — Streptococcal infections, dependent on type, may be highly infectious. Both asymptomatic carriers and those with active disease spread group A infection by airborne droplet transmission. Acquisition is followed by pharyngitis, follicular tonsillitis and cervical adenitis. Skin infection is facilitated by hyaluronidase which assists pyoderma to spread and involve deeper tissues, producing erysipelas and cellulitis. Erythema nodosum, and later rheumatic fever and glomerulonephritis, are immunological reactions to streptococcal infection. Neonates acquire group B streptococci from the birth canal and may develop septicemia (within 5 d) or later septicemia and meningitis.

Clinical features — **Erysipelas:** streptococcal invasion of the skin may result in a butterfly facial rash, (Figs 74 & 75) or a spreading eruption on the legs characterized by a red, swollen, painful epidermal lesion with a well demarcated raised edge. Bullae may form.

Pyoderma (Fig. 76): type 49 streptococci cause epidemics of skin sepsis with yellow crusts (with or without nephritis).

Ascending lymphangitis (Fig. 77): represents tender red inflamed lymph channels draining a streptococcal infection. Associated bacteremia may be a lethal complication.

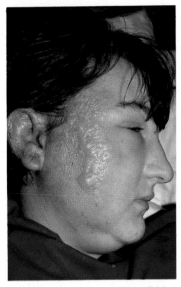

Fig. 74 Facial erysipelas with superficial bullae.

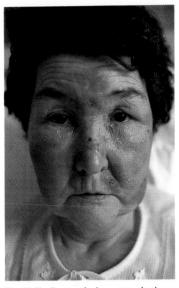

Fig. 75 Healing erysipelas: note raised edge.

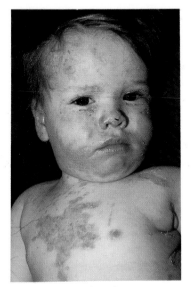

Fig. 76 Streptococcal pyoderma.

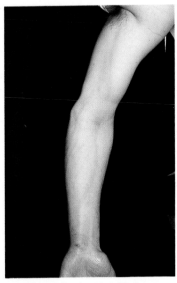

Fig. 77 Ascending lymphangitis from wound at wrist.

Clinical features
(contd)

Pharyngitis, tonsillitis and quinsy: after 2–4 d incubation, sore throat, fever, tachycardia and malaise are associated with pharyngitis or follicular tonsillitis (Fig. 78) and cervical adenitis. A bulging peritonsillar abscess (quinsy) may follow (Fig. 79). More rarely, suppurative adenitis, sinusitis, otitis media or mastoiditis develop. Viral pharyngitis, glandular fever and diphtheria must be differentiated.

Ludwig's angina (Fig. 80, p. 56): a synergistic infection involving oral microaerophilic streptococci in the submandibular space in which *Strep. pyogenes* may be present. May follow dental extraction in immunocompromised patients and can cause airways obstruction.

Henoch–Schöenlein purpura (Fig. 81, p. 56): affecting the buttocks and legs, and associated with arthritis and intestinal colic or bleeding. It is commonly related to streptococcal infection. Purpura is vascular in type: thrombocytopenia is absent.

Erythema nodosum (Fig. 82, p. 56): may complicate many acute infections, especially streptococcal or tuberculous, and sarcoidosis or drug therapy. Tender, red, raised lesions develop on the shins or elbows (p. 97).

Rheumatic fever: begins 2–3 wk after a streptococcal infection with fever, tachycardia, cardiac arrhythmias and murmurs, flitting large joint arthralgia, subcutaneous nodules and rashes, classically erythema marginatum (Fig. 83, p. 56). Two major or one major and two minor criteria with evidence of recent streptococcal disease confirm a diagnosis of rheumatic fever.

- *Major criteria*—carditis, polyarthritis, chorea, erythema marginatum, subcutaneous nodules.
- *Minor criteria*—fever, joint pain, high ESR or C-reactive protein, leucocytosis, prolonged P–R interval, past history of rheumatic fever.

The late cardiovascular sequelae of acute rheumatic fever include mitral and aortic valve disease with associated hemodynamic consequences.

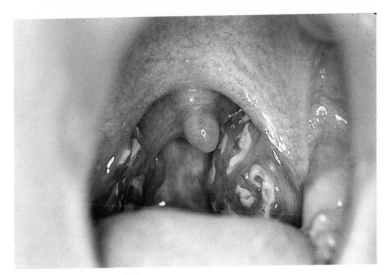

Fig. 78 Acute follicular tonsillitis.

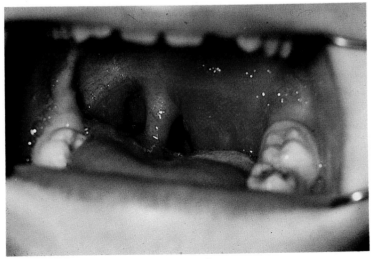

Fig. 79 Acute peritonsillar abscess (quinsy) with trismus.

Clinical features
(contd)

Glomerulonephritis: group A, type 12 or, during an epidemic of pyoderma, type 49 infections may be followed by fever, edema, hypertension and oliguria, proteinuria, hematuria and casts in the urine. Diagnosis of streptococcal infections requires isolation of streptococci from the throat, saliva or skin, or demonstration of a rising ASO titre. A polymorphonuclear leucocytosis and high ESR are usual.

Treatment

Penicillin G is advised initially but may be followed by oral penicillin V or amoxicillin in convalescence. Erythromycin is used in penicillin-allergic patients. To prevent recurrences of rheumatic fever, i.m. benzathine penicillin monthly (for unreliable patients especially) or oral penicillin V (or erythromycin) prophylaxis is used. High dose amoxicillin, clindamycin or erythromycin given immediately before dental surgery prevents *Strep. viridans* endocarditis in patients with rheumatic heart disease. High dose aspirin therapy has a beneficial effect on symptoms and outcome in acute rheumatic fever. Supportive treatment is necessary for cardiac dysfunction. Strict fluid and electrolyte balance plus protein restriction are essential in glomerulonephritis.

Prevention

Hospitalized patients should be isolated for 24–48 h, until chemotherapy renders them non-infectious. Eradication of streptococci from the pharynx requires 10-days therapy. Shorter courses encourage early relapse and risk of rheumatic fever.

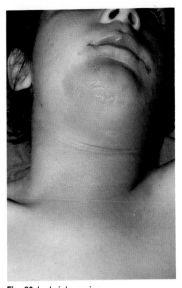

Fig. 80 Ludwig's angina.

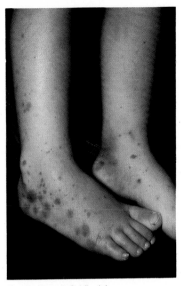

Fig. 81 Henoch-Schöenlein purpura.

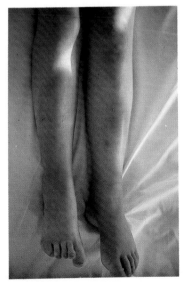

Fig. 82 Erythema nodosum.

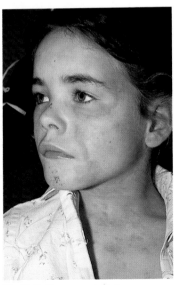

Fig. 83 Erythema marginatum.

21 / Scarlet fever

Etiology Beta-hemolytic streptococci of Lancefield's Group A elaborating erythrogenic toxin under the control of a lysogenic bacteriophage.

Incidence Worldwide distribution. Previously common, it is now rarely seen in the developed countries and is a milder disease than formerly.

Pathogenesis Both asymptomatic carriers and clinical cases disseminate streptococci, usually in airborne droplets. Wounds may also be a portal of entry. Scarlet fever results from absorption of erythrogenic toxin from the local infective site.

Clinical features The incubation period of 2–4 d is followed by the sudden onset of sore throat, fever, headache and often vomiting, contrasting with the slower onset of diphtheria and glandular fever. The tonsils are red and flecked with pus, and peritonsillar inflammation and edema may develop, associated with tender cervical adenitis. The tongue is initially furred and white (Fig. 84) and later smooth and red (Fig. 86). The rash consists of a scarlet blush (Fig. 85) with a punctate erythema, fading on pressure, which spares the circumoral region (Fig. 84). It peels after a few days (Fig. 86). Peripheral skin peeling is often marked on the palms and soles (Fig. 87). Streptococci isolated from throat swabs, a polymorphonuclear leucocytosis, and rising ASO and anti-DNAase B titres confirm the diagnosis.

Treatment Parenteral penicillin G followed by oral amoxicillin (or penicillin V). Erythromycin is substituted in penicillin-allergic patients.

Prevention Isolation is desirable in the acute phase. Penicillin therapy of contacts may limit institutional outbreaks.

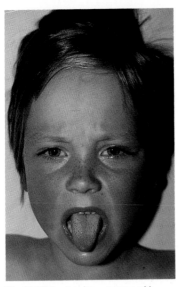

Fig. 84 White strawberry tongue with circumoral pallor.

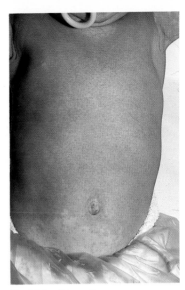

Fig. 85 Punctate erythema.

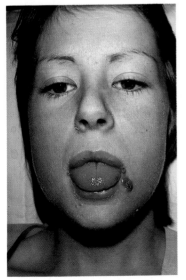

Fig. 86 Red strawberry tongue, perinasal peeling and herpes febrilis.

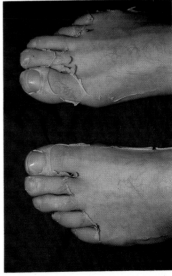

Fig. 87 Peripheral superficial skin peeling.

22 / Anthrax

Etiology	*Bacillus anthracis*, a Gram-positive sporing bacillus.
Incidence	Extremely rare in the US but more common in Europe and elsewhere due to animal enzootic disease.
Pathogenesis	A zoonosis acquired from contact with active cases among domestic mammals, including sheep, cattle and pigs, and with imported spore-infected hides, hair and unsterilized bone meal. Spores may be directly inoculated into the skin (cutaneous anthrax), inhaled (pulmonary anthrax) or, more rarely, ingested (intestinal anthrax).
Clinical features	**Cutaneous anthrax** (most common): a local papule at the site of inoculation develops into an ulcerated, necrotic, dark-centred eschar (malignant pustule: Figs 89 & 91), associated with extensive edema (Figs 88 & 90), regional adenitis and fever. **Pulmonary anthrax** (uncommon): severe disseminated hemorrhagic bronchopneumonia. Complicating septicemia is common. **Intestinal anthrax** (rare): varies from mild enteritis to a severe dysenteric illness. **Bacteremia**: from primary sites has a high mortality. Diagnosis is confirmed by isolation of *B. anthracis* from pustule, sputum, stools, blood or CSF.
Complications	• *Hemorrhagic pleuropericarditis.* • *Hemorrhagic meningitis.*
Treatment	Penicillin G (5–20 million units/d). Also erythromycin, tetracycline or chloramphenicol are effective alternative drugs. Antiserum therapy is no longer used.
Prevention	Not notifiable. A vaccine is available for those at risk of occupational exposure, e.g. professional gardeners (bone meal) and those handling imported hair and hides.

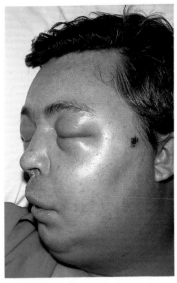

Fig. 88 Facial anthrax with massive edema gardener).

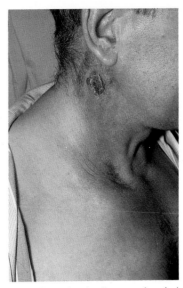

Fig. 89 Cervical eschar (bone meal worker).

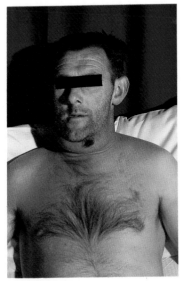

Fig. 90 Eschar and edema of neck and chest wall (farmer).

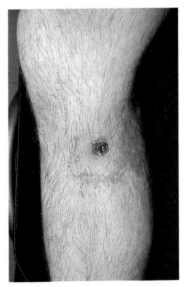

Fig. 91 Eschar on leg (bone meal worker).

23 / Diphtheria

Etiology	Toxigenic *Corynebacterium diphtheriae*, a Gram-positive bacillus. Toxin production is determined by a lysogenic bacteriophage.
Incidence	Worldwide distribution: diphtheria is rare where there is a high rate of immunization.
Pathogenesis	Airborne droplet transmission from active cases. *C. diphtheriae* multiplies in the upper airways and forms an adherent membrane of bacteria, WBC and necrotic tissue. There is associated edema of the neck. Laryngeal obstruction can occur in infants. Absorption of a potent toxin causes later cardiac and neurological complications. It becomes fixed to these tissues, disrupting protein synthesis and causing demyelination.
Clinical features	The incubation period of 2–4 d is followed by fever, disproportionate tachycardia, malaise, headache and symptoms at the site of invasion—nose, tonsils, pharynx or larynx (Figs 92 & 93). Typical adherent membrane appears on mucosa (Fig. 93), associated with lymphadenopathy and surrounding edema (bull-neck appearance). Stridor may be present in infants with laryngeal diphtheria. Diphtheria toxin causes cardiac arrhythmias, conduction defects and failure 1–3 wk after onset and, later, peripheral neuropathies. These include palatal, ocular, diaphragmatic (phrenic nerve) and late-onset limb pareses, 3–10 wk after onset. Diagnosis is confirmed by isolation of *C. diphtheriae* (Fig. 94) from throat swabs and tests for toxin production (Elek method).
Treatment	Treatment must not be delayed pending laboratory confirmation. 10 to 60 000 units of antitoxin are given intravenously if a diluted intradermal test dose shows no significant reaction. Penicillin G or erythromycin should be prescribed. Tracheostomy is rarely indicated.
Prevention	Notifiable: strict isolation is mandatory. Routine immunization (toxoid vaccine) is given in infancy. Carriers should be treated with erythromycin.

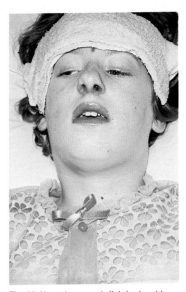

Fig. 92 Nasopharyngeal diphtheria with bloody discharge and bull neck.

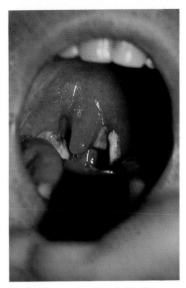

Fig. 93 Pharyngotonsillar diphtheria: note adherent membrane with curled edge.

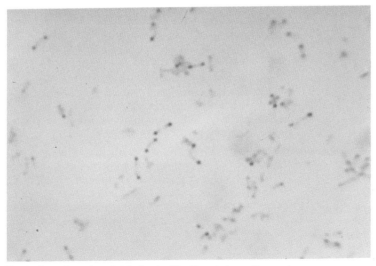

Fig. 94 *Corynebacterium diphtheriae*: bacilli with metachromatic granules.

24 / Tetanus

Etiology *Clostridium tetani,* an anaerobic, Gram-positive sporing bacillus.

Incidence Worldwide distribution: more common where there is no immunization, and in farming communities.

Pathogenesis *Cl. tetani* is an environmental organism which is introduced into deep traumatic anaerobic wounds or into the umbilical stump in neonates. Vegetative multiplication and toxin elaboration follow. Two toxins are produced:

- *Tetanolysin*—causes labile hypertension, arrhythmias, vasoconstriction and sweating.
- *Tetanospasmin*—fixes to nuclei of motor nerves and neuromuscular end-plates causing muscle spasm.

Clinical features The incubation period is usually 5–14 d, dependent on the size and site of the inoculum. Cephalic tetanus has a short incubation and poor prognosis. The onset of muscular spasm and rigidity is insidious and characterized by trismus, risus sardonicus and, later, opisthotonos (Fig. 95). Spasms are triggered by noise, lights or movement. Consciousness and sensation are unimpaired. Respiratory arrest or asphyxia may occur. Neonatal tetanus begins 3–10 d after birth and has a very poor prognosis (Fig. 96).

Treatment Mainly supportive. Muscular spasms are controlled with intravenous diazepam. Therapeutic paralysis and IPPV are infrequently required. Human tetanus immunoglobulin (30 iu/kg; iu = international units) and i.v. or i.m. penicillin G should be administered.

Prevention Notifiable. Traumatic wounds must be thoroughly cleansed. Toxoid vaccine and human tetanus immunoglobulin should be given as required. All infants should be routinely immunized. Non-immune mothers can be immunized before delivery. Infection does not confer immunity: immunization is required on convalescence.

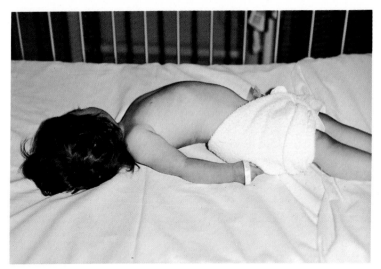

Fig. 95 Tetanic spasm (opisthotonos).

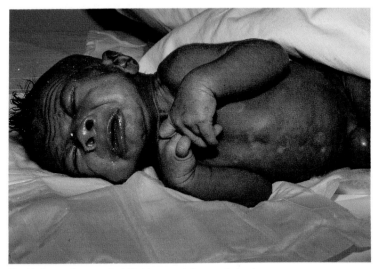

Fig. 96 Neonatal tetanus (wrinkled brow and risus sardonicus).

25 / Enteric (typhoid and paratyphoid) fevers

Etiology	*Salmonella typhi, Salmonella paratyphi* A and B.
Incidence	Worldwide distribution: more common in tropics and where poor hygiene/sanitation prevail.
Pathogenesis	Fecal–oral transmission via contact and contamination of water and food. Ingested *S. typhi* not killed by gastric acid, enter the ileum, invade lymphatics and multiply in the reticuloendothelial system. Subsequent bacteremia and gut re-invasion cause the clinical illness.
Clinical features	The initial bacteremic phase, lasting about 1 wk, is characterized by a step-wise rise in fever, relative bradycardia, constipation, splenomegaly, increasing confusion and, less commonly, a pink macular (rose spot) truncal rash (Fig. 97). Untreated, the patient then deteriorates with increasing toxemia, dehydration, a maintained fever, and abdominal cramps and diarrhea (Fig. 98). Recovery usually commences in the third week but relapse and intestinal perforation or hemorrhage may occur. Diagnosis is confirmed by blood and stool cultures, and a specific 'O' antibody response in the Widal test. Stools often remain positive for several weeks: long-term carriage occurs in less than 5%.
Treatment	The antibiotics of choice are now ciprofloxacin, chloramphenicol, trimethoprim–sulfamethoxazole and amoxicillin. Fluid and electrolyte balance are strictly monitored. Ciprofloxacin eradicates chronic carriage in >80%: cholecystectomy cures 75% if gallstones are present.
Prevention	Notifiable: strict isolation is necessary. Good hygiene/ sewage disposal and clean water supplies are essential. Monovalent typhoid vaccine gives partial protection for 3 yr.

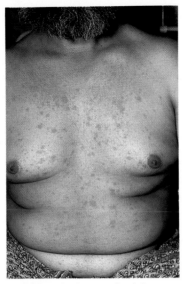

Fig. 97 Extensive 'rose spot' rash in paratyphoid A.

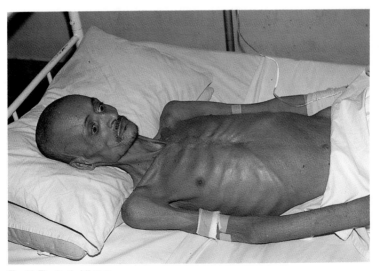

Fig. 98 The 'typhoid' state.

26 / Infantile gastroenteritis

Etiology   Usually viral, due to rotavirus (30%) or other small round viruses (astroviruses and caliciviruses) and enteroviruses, but may also be due to enteropathogenic *Escherichia coli* (EPEC) serotypes (0111, 0128, 0142, etc.) and *Salmonella, Shigella* or *Campylobacter* species. *Cryptosporidium* infection may also be responsible. In a third no etiological agent is identified.

Incidence   Diarrheal illness is among the most common causes of morbidity and hospital admission in infants. It is responsible for up to 25% of infant morbidity in some developing countries and in such areas is the most common cause of death in infancy.

Pathogenesis   Acquisition follows fecal–oral transmission from acute cases (viruses, shigella, EPEC), via foodstuffs or milk/water (salmonellosis, campylobacteriosis) or from carriers (salmonellosis). *Cryptosporidium* may spread via water or from animals. Enteritis is caused by either gut wall invasion and inflammation (e.g. shigellosis and salmonellosis), adherence and cytotoxity (e.g. rotavirus and EPEC enteritis), or invasion of the gut wall plus enterotoxin production (e.g. campylobacteriosis).

Clinical features   The cardinal features are diarrhea and vomiting, which vary from trivial to profuse. Blood staining of feces is more typical of invasive disease due to bacteria, especially shigellosis and campylobacterosis. Fluid loss may cause dehydration, hypovolemia and hypotension (Figs 99, 100 & 101). Excoriation of the buttocks and perineum may occur (Fig. 102). Bacteremia may accompany salmonellosis and EPEC enteritis. *Esch. coli* 0157 is associated with verotoxin production and may cause hemolytic–uremic syndrome (and hemorrhagic colitis in adults).

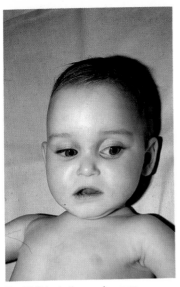

Fig. 99 Dehydration: sunken eyes, corrugated axillary folds and dry mouth.

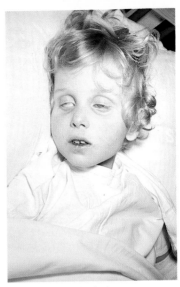

Fig. 100 Severe dehydration.

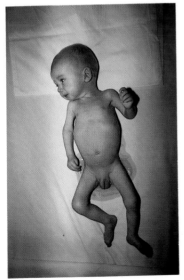

Fig. 101 Dehydrated infant; clear fluid stool after glucose/electrolyte feed.

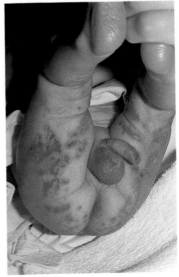

Fig. 102 Excoriation of buttocks and perineum.

Clinical features
(contd)

Bacteremia may accompany salmonellosis and EPEC enteritis but is uncommon with other bacterial diarrheas. Diagnosis requires stool and, where relevant, blood cultures. Enteropathogenic viruses in stools may be demonstrated by electron microscopy (Fig. 103) or polyacrilamide gel electrophoresis.

Complications

Hypernatremia: was most commonly associated with the use of hypertonic milk feeds (no longer marketed) during early disease and was associated, in severe cases, with intracranial sinus thrombosis, secondary cerebral edema causing focal or generalized convulsions and neurological defects, and renal thrombosis/necrosis (Fig. 104).

Acute colitis: can follow salmonellosis or campylobacterosis but is unusual in children.

Lactose intolerance: transient secondary disaccharidase deficiency can follow rotavirus or EPEC enteritis. It usually settles within 2 mth, and requires substitution of non-lactose containing milks.

Hemolytic-uremic syndrome (Esch. coli 0157): presents with a microangiopathic anemia, thrombocytopenia and renal failure.

Treatment

Rehydration using oral or parenteral glucose-electrolyte solutions (i.e. Pedialyte or Lytien), followed by reintroduction of graduated, increasing strength milk feeds over 3–4 d. Antibiotics are contraindicated except in bacteremic infants. Hemolytic–uremic syndrome may require transfusion and dialysis.

Prevention

Many forms notifiable (e.g. salmonellosis). Hospitalized cases must be strictly isolated. General preventive measures include food hygiene precautions, aseptic preparation of milk feeds, adequate cooking of contaminated meats, e.g. poultry, encouragement of breast feeding and, notably in developing countries, the provision of clean water supplies and effective sanitation. Rotavirus and other vaccines are under development.

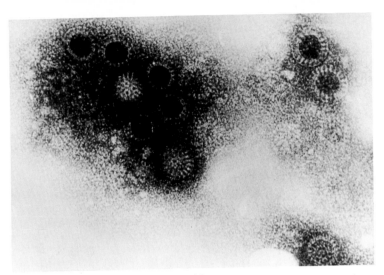

Fig. 103 Electron micrograph of rotavirus particles.

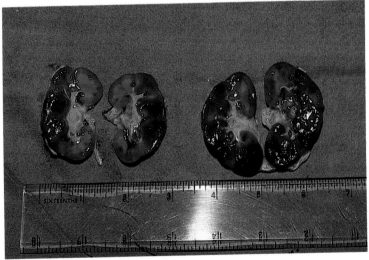

Fig. 104 Bilateral renal thrombosis in dehydrated neonate.

27 / **Pseudomembranous colitis**

Etiology Enterotoxin-producing *Clostridium difficile*, a Gram-positive sporing anaerobe.

Incidence Rare, but may occur in sub-epidemic form in surgical wards. It affects up to 3% of patients receiving clindamycin but may occur after any antibiotic therapy, sometimes up to 6 wk later.

Pathogenesis Colonic overgrowth of *Cl. difficile* induced by antibiotic exposure, followed by enterotoxin production and mucosal damage typified by summit lesions on colonic mucosa (Fig. 105), glandular disruption, epithelial necrosis and focal inflammation. Macroscopic colonic pseudomembranes are present (Fig. 106). Most commonly follows broad spectrum antibiotic exposure but classically associated with clindamycin. The source of *Cl. difficile* may be hospital cross-infection.

Clinical features • *Mild*—slight persistent diarrhea, self-limiting within 2 wk in 80%.
• *Severe*—frequent bloody diarrhea with abdominal and rectal tenesmus associated with fever and dehydration, which may progress to toxic dilatation (Fig. 107), perforation of colon and death. Can present during treatment or for several weeks thereafter.

Diagnosis is substantiated by sigmoidoscopy, rectal biopsy and examination of stools for *Cl. difficile* and enterotoxin.

Treatment Vancomycin 125 mg, q 6–8 h, by mouth for 7–10 d. Response is usually rapid but up to 10% of patients relapse and require a longer treatment duration. Oral metronidazole is also a useful regimen.

Prevention Not notifiable: known cases must be isolated to prevent cross-colonization of other patients. Instruments and endoscopes used rectally should be sterilized with sporicidal disinfectants.

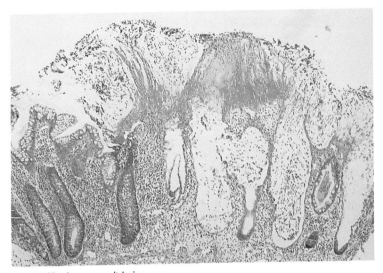

Fig. 105 Histology: summit lesion.

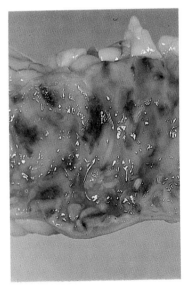

Fig. 106 Colonic pseudomembranes.

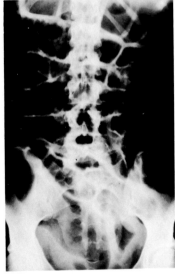

Fig. 107 Toxic dilatation of colon (precolectomy).

28 / Meningococcal infections

Etiology	*Neisseria meningitidis*: a capsulated Gram-negative diplococcus. Epidemics are due to types A, B and C and sporadic cases are usually caused by types B, W135 and other serotypes.
Incidence	Epidemic fluctuation: up to 3000 sporadic cases per year in the US. Secondary cases may occur in close family and nursery school contacts.
Pathogenesis	Spread occurs via airborne droplet transmission from nasopharynx of cases and carriers. Subsequent fulminating bacteremia or subacute bacteremia and meningitis commonly follow, but many acquire asymptomatic nasopharyngeal carriage. In acute cases endotoxin release from intact *N. meningitidis* causes antibody-independent complement activation, shock, disseminated intravascular coagulation and generalized Schwartzman reaction (capillary damage, thrombosis and hemorrhage into skin and adrenals). Immune complex deposition disease may cause arthritis.
Clinical features	**Fulminating meningococcemia:** overwhelming shock, petechiae and ecchymoses (Figs 108, 109, 110 & 111) and adrenal infarction (Fig. 112, p. 76) (Waterhouse-Friderichsen syndrome); death usually occurs within 6–18 h (Fig. 113, p. 76). Most common in infants.
	Bacterial meningitis: severe toxemia, meningeal irritation and petechial rash (not always present) associated with a polymorphonuclear CSF pleocytosis (plus low CSF sugar and elevated protein). Usually fatal within 24–72 h if untreated. More common in older children and young adults.
	Recurrent meningitis: associated with antibody and late-acting complement component deficiences (rare).
	Pneumonia: uncommon.
	Diagnosis is established by isolation of *N. meningitidis* from CSF and blood cultures or by antigen detection.

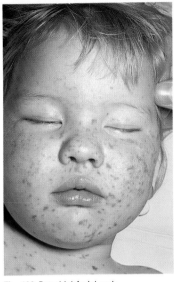

Fig. 108 Petechial facial rash.

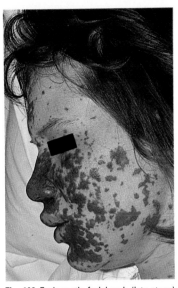

Fig. 109 Ecchymotic facial rash (late stage).

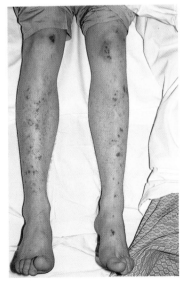

Fig. 110 Hemorrhagic rash (adult with meningitis).

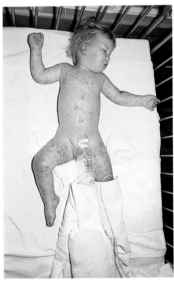

Fig. 111 Waterhouse–Friderichsen syndrome.

Complications *Immune complex arthritis* and *pericarditis* can arise 1 wk or more after onset. Extensive skin necrosis may follow ecchymotic hemorrhage. Later renal tubular damage in cases surviving severe disease.

Treatment Intravenous penicillin G 300 000 units/kg/24 h in 6 divided doses. For children older than 1 mth to up to 12 yr, 100 000 to 300 000 units/kg/d in divided doses every 4–6 h. Intrathecal therapy is unnecessary. Chloramphenicol should be used for penicillin-allergic patients. Steroids, except in massive doses for Waterhouse–Friderichsen syndrome, are of little benefit. Monoclonal antibodies against endotoxin and tumour necrosis factor may prove of benefit in the future. Rifampin is used to eradicate persistent nasopharyngeal carriage in patients following penicillin treatment.

Prevention Notifiable: strict isolation is necessary, but cases among hospital contacts are extremely rare.

Chemoprophylaxis: close family and nursery school contacts should receive rifampin (5 mg/kg, 12-hourly) plus, in adults, minocycline (100 mg, 12-hourly) for 2 d. Hospital contacts are not usually at risk. Secondary cases are most likely to occur within 24 h of the index case: chemoprophylaxis should therefore be started immediately. Ciprofloxacin (single-dose) may supersede rifampin as the agent of choice. Meningococci may persist after penicillin treatment and cases should receive prophylactic antibiotics to protect subsequent contacts.

Immunoprophylaxis: a vaccine is available for types A and C and is likely to become generally used, either for control of epidemics, e.g. recent outbreaks in West Africa and at the Haj in Mecca, or individual protection of contacts (together with chemoprophylaxis as above).

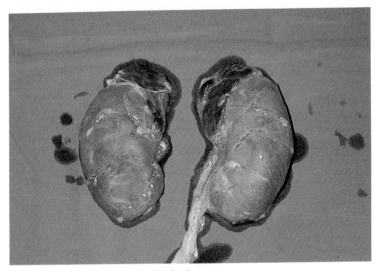

Fig. 112 Bilateral hemorrhagic adrenal infarction.

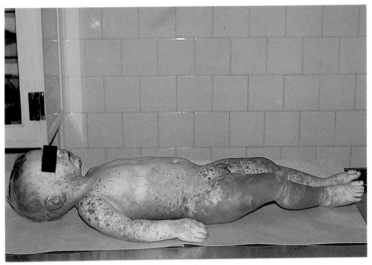

Fig. 113 Death from Waterhouse–Friderichsen syndrome.

29 / Bacterial (pyogenic) meningitis

Etiology
: *N. meningitidis*, Pittman type, B, *H. influenzae* (HIB) and *Streptococcus pneumoniae*.

Incidence
: 15 000 cases/yr in the US: *N. meningitidis* 50%.

Pathogenesis
: • *Strep. pneumoniae*—usually endogenous. May invade meninges via blood stream, sinuses, middle ear infections or basal fractures.
: • *HIB*—an exogenous infection acquired from carriers of the virulent serotype.
: • *N. meningitidis*—(see p. 73).

  Pathology is characterized by acute inflammatory infiltration of meninges and ependyma of ventricles.

Clinical features
: A severe, acute onset illness, characterized within 24–48 h by high fever, headache, neck stiffness (Fig. 114), photophobia, vomiting and confusion. Focal CNS signs and coma indicate a poor prognosis. The meningococcal rash (p. 74) is typical: very rarely seen with other forms. Diagnosis is by CSF examination (polymorph pleocytosis, low sugar) and isolation of the pathogen from CSF and blood cultures.

Complications
: • *Persistent fever*—often due to drugs.
: • *Intracranial abscess* (rare).
: • *Sterile subdural effusions* (rare).
: • *CNS abnormalities*—decerebrate rigidity (Fig. 115), hydrocephalus, deafness, epilepsy.
: • *Immune-complex arthritis* (meningococcal).
: • *Septic arthritis*.

Treatment
: • *Meningococcal and pneumococcal meningitis*—penicillin G (see p. 75, meningococcal infections).
: • *HIB and undiagnosed bacterial meningitis.* Chloramphenicol 80 mg/kg/d in divided doses q 6 h with up to 100 mg/kg required to achieve adequate CSF concentrations. Ceftriaxone dosing in children is 100 mg/kg once a day or in divided doses q 12 h; dosing in adults is 2 g q 12–24 h. Cefotaxime dosing for serious infections in adults is 6–12 g/d; dosing in children is 150 mg/kg/d as q 4–6 h.

Prevention
: Notifiable: isolation of meningococcal infection. Meningococcal and HIB vaccines are available. Rifampin for HIB and meningococcal contacts.

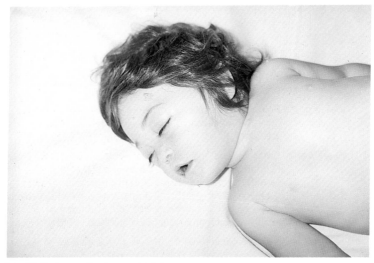

Fig. 114 Neck retraction (severe rigidity).

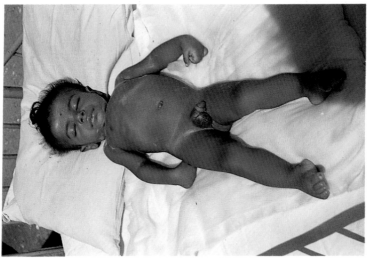

Fig. 115 Decerebrate state (*H. influenzae meningitis*).

30 / **Viral meningitis**

Etiology	Enteroviruses (echovirus, Coxsackie virus, poliovirus), mumps virus, herpes simplex viruses-1/2.
Incidence	Epidemic fluctuations in incidence, enteroviruses in most summers and mumps every 3–4 yr. High incidence of asymptomatic infection.
Pathogenesis	Enteroviruses spread via fecal–oral route, most common in young children who transmit infection to older family contacts. Mumps infection spreads by droplet airborne transmission from active cases. Both cause lymphocytic meningitis with minimal brain and spinal parenchymal inflammation. Encephalitis is rare.
Clinical features	• *Enteroviruses* cause a biphasic illness, initially mild prodromal febrile URTI or enteritis followed by recrudescent fever, positional headache, neck and spinal rigidity (Fig. 116), photophobia, vomiting and, in some, a maculopapular rash (Fig. 117) and pharyngitis or conjunctivitis. The patient is usually not very ill.
	• *Mumps meningitis* causes similar signs of meningeal irritation, usually, but not invariably, preceded by salivary gland involvement (p. 9).
Complications	Echo and Coxsackie viruses rarely cause an *ascending paralysis* similar to poliomyelitis. Mumps may be complicated by orchitis, oophoritis, pancreatitis or arthritis.
Treatment	Analgesia, antiemetics and several days bed rest are required.
Prevention	Poliovirus infections are notifiable: all cases require strict isolation. Poliovaccine is type specific and has no protective effect against other enteroviruses. Echo and Coxsackie virus vaccines are not available. Mumps vaccine is widely available both alone and as combined MMR vaccine (p. 9).

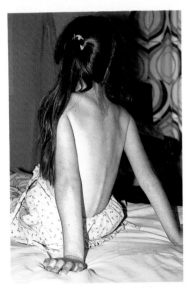

Fig. 116 Tripod sign of spinal rigidity.

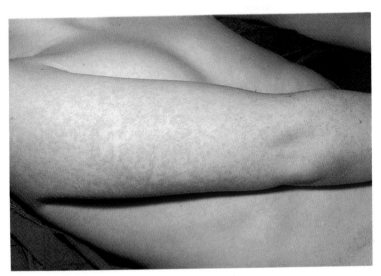

Fig. 117 Enteroviral rash.

31 / Primary tuberculosis

Etiology	*Mycobacterium tuberculosis* (human and bovine).
Incidence	Remains a major health care problem worldwide, Incidence is increasing in the US, especially among high-risk groups such as drug addicts, HIV positive, and the homeless.
Pathogenesis	**Human tuberculosis:** airborne droplet transmission from active pulmonary cases. Inhalation is followed by formation of sub-pleural (Ghon) focus and hilar gland involvement (primary complex) which usually heals but may rupture into bronchus, pleura or pulmonary vessels followed by local, pleural, pericardial, bronchial or hematogenous spread.

Bovine tuberculosis: spread by infected milk, may cause primary tonsillar infection with associated cervical gland involvement. These glands may caseate and form sinuses in the neck. Bowel involvement may cause later tuberculous peritonitis.

Clinical features and complications

Asymptomatic infection with healing: Mantoux becomes positive in 6–8 wk. Primary hilar gland(s) may be obvious on chest X-ray at that time (Fig. 118). The tendency of such lesions is to heal but later reactivation may occur (see *Late complications,* p. 83). Primary infection may be associated with immunological hypersensitivity phenomena including erythema nodosum (see p. 97) and phlyctenular conjunctivitis.

Tuberculous pleural effusion: secondary to rupture of hilar glands into the pleural cavity, can fill the hemithorax (Fig. 119). Tubercle bacilli are present in effusion fluid.

Miliary tuberculosis: miliary pulmonary infiltration with widespread dissemination and foci of infection including tuberculous meningitis follows bloodstream invasion. The chest X-ray usually has a characteristic 'snowstorm' appearance (Fig. 120). Choroidal tubercles may be present on fundoscopy (Fig. 121). Tubercle bacilli may be cultured from CSF and urine, but only exceptionally rarely from blood.

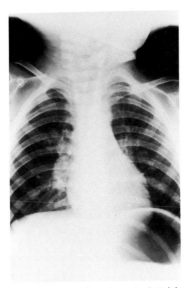

Fig. 118 Primary tuberculous gland at right hilum.

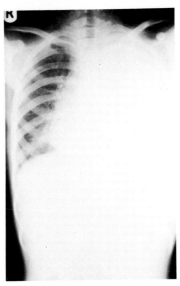

Fig. 119 Primary tuberculous pleural effusion.

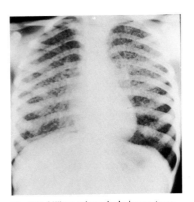

Fig. 120 Miliary tuberculosis (snowstorm appearance).

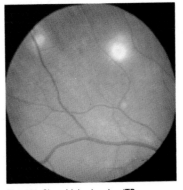

Fig. 121 Choroidal tubercles (TB meningitis) in fundus oculi.

Clinical features and complications (contd) **Tuberculous bronchopneumonia:** either localized to a segment (epituberculosis) or widespread throughout both lungs (Fig. 122). Can result in rapid weight loss and death within months (galloping consumption).

Late complications: tuberculous pericarditis, tuberculous osteitis and arthritis (after 5–10 yr) (Fig. 123), renal tuberculosis (after 10–15 yr), reactivation of pulmonary disease in adulthood (Fig. 124). Late pericardial involvement may cause calcification of pericardium and constrictive pericarditis.

Tuberculosis and AIDS: both classical and atypical (*Myco. avium-intracellulare* complex—MAC) infections are common in AIDS patients (Topic 43) and are commonly multidrug-resistant.

Treatment Triple therapy: rifampin, ethambutol and isoniazid. Pyrazinamide is often added in patients with tuberculous meningitis. Severely ill children and many with tuberculous meningitis require steroid therapy. Asymptomatic infections in contacts require isoniazid and rifampin therapy (if X-ray abnormal) or prophylactic isoniazid (if X-ray remains normal).

Prevention Notifiable: isolation is necessary until effective chemotherapy has rendered respiratory secretions and urine non-infective (usually days to weeks). All close contacts should be screened to detect the source of infection (usually a family member) and other early cases, notably among siblings. Those converting to Mantoux positivity require follow-up chest X-ray and, in many cases, antituberculous chemotherapy (see above). New immigrants from endemic areas with respiratory symptoms require a diagnostic chest X-ray.

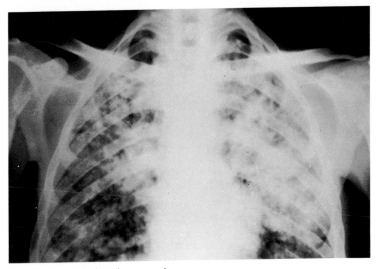

Fig. 122 Tuberculous bronchopneumonia.

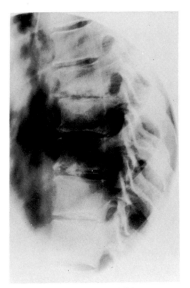

Fig. 123 Tuberculous spondylitis: note erosion of vertebral bodies (Pott's disease).

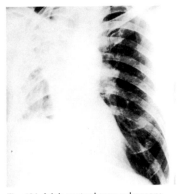

Fig. 124 Adult post-primary pulmonary tuberculosis (healed fibrotic disease).

32 / Pertussis (whooping cough)

Etiology	*Bordetella pertussis*, a Gram-negative bacillus.
Incidence	Sporadic disease, subject to epidemic variation every 3–5 yr.
Pathogenesis	Airborne droplet transmission from active cases. Inflammatory bronchitis is accompanied by mucosal necrosis and mucus hypersecretion, peribronchial infiltration and, in many cases, plugging of airways and absorption collapse.
Clinical features	The incubation period of about 5–10 d is followed by upper respiratory catarrh, lasting for about a week. The paroxysmal cough then develops, accompanied by terminal inspiratory whoop and persists for several weeks. Cough may cause cyanosis, vomiting and transient apnea. Chest examination is usually normal between paroxysms. Diagnosis may be confirmed by culture of nasopharyngeal swabs on selective media in early disease and by serology. An absolute lymphocytosis is typically present.
Complications	• *Respiratory*—secondary bacterial bronchopneumonia, segmental/lobar/pulmonary collapse secondary to aspiration (Figs 125 & 126), bronchiectasis. • *Neurological*—a rare encephalopathy is characterized by convulsions, coma and progressive CNS signs. • *Pressure-related*—paroxysmal cough may cause subconjunctival hemorrhage (Fig. 127), skin petechiae, hernia and rectal prolapse.
Treatment	Oral erythromycin 50 mg/kg/d (maximum 2 g/d) in two doses × 14 d may attenuate severity.
Prevention	Notifiable: isolate hospitalized cases. Polyvalent whole-cell derived agglutinogen (DTP or single) vaccine gives 95% protection. Erythromycin within 5 d of contact may prevent disease.

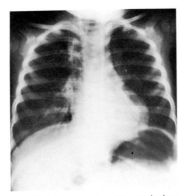

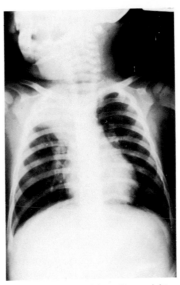

Fig. 125 Left lower lobe collapse: shadow behind the heart.

Fig. 126 Right upper lobe collapse: right apex.

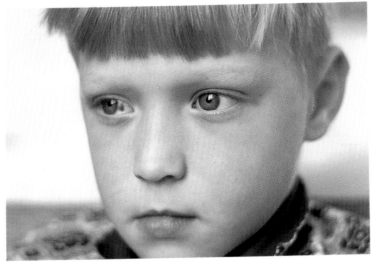

Fig. 127 Subconjunctival hemorrhage.

33 / Acute croup and bronchiolitis

Etiology
Para-influenza (croup) and respiratory syncytial virus (bronchiolitis).

Incidence
Acute croup usually affects children from 3 to 36 mth: bronchiolitis—infants less than 3 mth. Both are cold weather illnesses and are distributed worldwide.

Pathogenesis
Spread by airborne droplet transmission from active cases. In croup, edema and inflammatory narrowing of upper airways result in stridor and hoarseness. Bronchiolitis is associated with necrosis, paralysis of cilia and mucus plugging of terminal airways. Secondary bacterial infection may cause bronchopneumonia.

Clinical features
Croup: mild fever and coryza are followed by barking cough, hoarseness, inspiratory stridor and increasing respiratory distress always worse at night.

Bronchiolitis: the baby may be afebrile but is distressed with nasal flare, tracheal tug, cough, subcostal and intercostal recession, crepitations and rhonchi. Dyspnea prevents feeding, leading to dehydration.

The chest X-ray may be clear or show peribronchitis (Fig. 128) or bronchopneumonia. Cardiac failure may occur in very young infants. Diagnosis is achieved by examination of nasopharyngeal secretions by fluorescent antibody and tissue culture methods.

Treatment
Severely ill cases are treated with oxygen-enriched, humidified air. Severe croup requires use of i.v. hydrocortisone to clear the edematous airway: tracheostomy is rarely necessary. Babies with bronchiolitis may need antibiotics (such as erythromycin), bronchodilators, i.v. fluids and hydrocortisone in severe cases. Aerosolized ribavirin may be useful for severe RSV infections

Prevention
No vaccines are currently available.

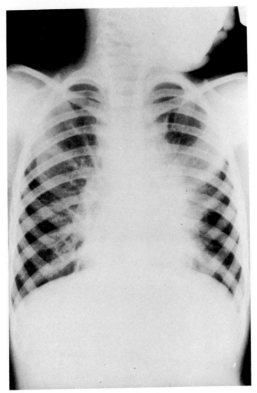

Fig. 128 Diffuse peribronchial infiltration.

34 / **Legionnaires' disease**

Etiology	*Legionella pneumophila* and other species: small Gram-negative coccobacilli.
Incidence	May account for 3–5% of atypical pneumonias. Sporadic incidence is intermixed with common-source outbreaks in hotels and hospitals.
Pathogenesis	Legionellae are environmental organisms which become established in warm water environments, e.g. air conditioning and shower systems, and jacuzzis. Point-source outbreaks are common. Aerosols probably account for inhalational acquisition by most patients. Multisystem infection follows, associated with severe bronchiolopneumonitis. Renal failure and CNS involvement may be severe.
Clinical features	The incubation period of 2–10 d is followed by malaise, fever, myalgia, rigors, headache and diarrhea. Mental confusion is prominent. Failure of empirical penicillin therapy is typical. Dry cough develops but other respiratory signs may be minimal. Several days later, crepitations may be heard but consolidation is often absent. Chest X-ray shows lobar or diffuse infiltration (Fig. 129): an effusion may be present. Early diagnosis can be achieved by antigen detection in urine or biopsy of bronchial or lung tissue. Serological tests (IFAT) confirm the diagnosis. Untreated disease may last 2–3 wk.
Complications	Renal and respiratory failure, and cerebellar ataxia may occur. The mortality is about 10%.
Treatment	Intravenous erythromycin is the drug of choice. Rifampin or ciprofloxacin are added in non-responding patients.
Prevention	Notifiable. Case-to-case transmission does not occur: isolation is not necessary. Infected water systems should be adequately and, if necessary, repeatedly chlorinated.

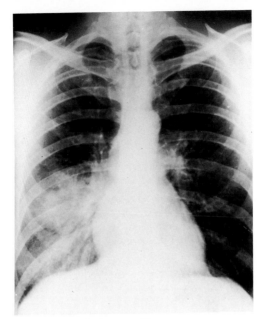

Fig. 129 Legionnaires' pneumonitis.

35 / Atypical pneumonia

Etiology
: *Mycoplasma pneumoniae, Chlamydia psittaci, Chlamydia pneumoniae,* and *Coxiella burnetii.*

Incidence
: *M. pneumoniae* and *Chl. pneumoniae* pneumonia are more common in young people. Psittacosis is acquired from birds (e.g. parrots, budgies and pigeons) and is seen in fanciers and handlers. *C. burnetii* (Q-fever) is a disease of sheep, goats and cattle, occasionally seen in vets and farmers.

Pathogenesis
: The pathogen is usually inhaled by droplet emission from active cases (*M. pneumoniae*) or aerosol/dust from contaminated environments (psittacosis/Q-fever). All cause pneumonitis.

Clinical features
: These diseases have an incubation period of 1–3 wk and a subacute onset. Prodromal features may include fever, rigors, myalgia and arthralgia, anorexia, vomiting, diarrhea and pharyngitis. These are followed by dry cough, associated with a mild pneumonitis which can be patchy, multifocal or perihilar (Figs 130 & 131). Occasionally severe pneumonia can occur. Signs of consolidation are often absent. The illness may last for 2–3 wk and the diagnosis is established serologically.

Complications
: **Mycoplasma pneumonitis:** arthritis, hemolysis, encephalitis and Stevens–Johnson syndrome (p. 99).
  Q-fever: endocarditis and liver involvement (likely if phase I antibody persists).
  Psittacosis: renal failure, encephalitis, endocarditis and DIC.

Treatment
: Erythromycin is the drug of choice for *M. pneumoniae* and *Chl. pneumoniae* infections. In adults, tetracycline is preferred for Q-fever and psittacosis.

Prevention
: Avoidance of exposure, and hygiene measures in bird and animal husbandry. Experimental vaccines are not generally applicable. Routine isolation of active cases is not necessary.

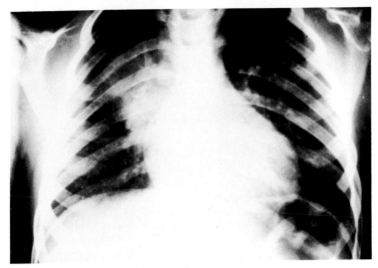

Fig. 130 *Mycoplasma pneumoniae* pneumonia.

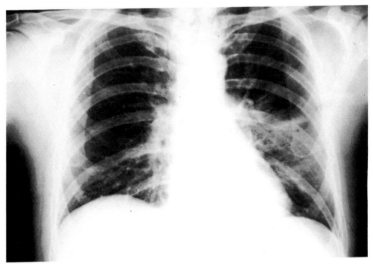

Fig. 131 Psittacosis pneumonitis (hazy left mid-zone infiltration).

36 / Bacterial pneumonia

Etiology Lobar pneumonia is usually caused by *Strep. pneumoniae* and bronchopneumonia additionally by *Staph. aureus,* and *H. influenzae.* Primary Gram-negative pneumonia is rare.

Incidence Usually sporadic but hospital outbreaks may be caused by Gram-negative pathogens.

Pathogenesis Pneumococcal pneumonia is an endogenous infection. Severe disease can occur in alcoholics and in splenectomized, immunocompromised (AIDS) and sickle cell anemia patients. Staphylococcal infections may complicate influenza and other viral URTI. *H. influenzae* pneumonia occurs in children or in chronic bronchitics. Gram-negative bacilli, e.g. *Esch. coli; Klebsiella* spp. and *P. aeruginosa,* cause opportunistic infections, notably in neutropenic cancer patients. *Klebsiella* spp. pneumonia may occur in the elderly.

Clinical features Range from localized consolidation, toxemia and fever to severe bacteremic disease with local and systemic complications, and shock (Gram-negative infections). Chest X-ray demonstrates lobar consolidation (Fig. 132) or multifocal opacification. Pathogens can be isolated from sputum, blood and tissue cultures. Pneumococcal antigen is present in sputum and urine.

Complications Include *lung abscess* (p. 95) *empyema, bacteremia, meningitis* (usually Gram-negative infections) and other *metastatic disease.*

Treatment
• *Strep. pneumoniae*—penicillin G or V.
• *H. influenzae*—amoxicillin, parenteral ceftriaxone.
• *Staph. aureus*—oxacillin, clindamycin or an antistaphylococcal cephalosporin are alternatives.
• *Gram-negative infections*—gentamicin or ciprofloxacin plus, in immunocompromised patients, piperacillin.
• Severe community-acquired pneumonia—cefuroxime or ceftriaxone plus erythromycin.

Resistance may influence future choice of antibiotic(s).

Prevention Polyvalent pneumococcal vaccine (Pneumovax) for predisposed patients, e.g. sickle cell disease, post-splenectomy and severe bronchitics.

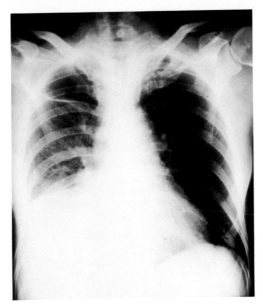

Fig. 132 Pneumococcal lobar pneumonia.

37 / Lung abscess

Etiology *Strep. pneumoniae* (post-pneumonic), oral anaerobes (post-aspiration), *Staph. aureus* (post-pneumonic), mixed flora (post-embolic abscess).

Incidence A sporadic endogenous infection.

Pathogenesis May complicate primary pneumonia (pneumococci, staphylococci and Gram-negative bacilli), lobar collapse, aspiration of oral secretions (alcoholic, epileptic, comatose or ventilated patients), pulmonary infarction and tricuspid endocarditis (usually *Staph. aureus* in drug addicts).

Clinical features May present as: a complication of known pneumonia, unexplained fever in comatose or ventilated patients, a recurrence of fever in patients with pulmonary embolism or tricuspid endocarditis, hemoptysis and fever, or pyrexia of unknown origin.

Physical signs can be minimal in the absence of overlying pleurisy or complicating empyema. Foul sputum usually indicates anaerobic infection. Chest X-ray is usually diagnostic (Fig. 133). Blood and sputum cultures are mandatory.

Treatment Prolonged antibiotic courses of 6–8 wk are usually required. Post-pneumonic and aspiration abscess should be treated with penicillin G plus metronidazole (or clindamycin). Staphylococcal lung abscesses require oxacillin or clindamycin. Alternative therapy is with an antistaphylococcal cephalosporin. Complicating empyema must be repeatedly aspirated or surgically drained.

Prevention Important factors include adequate therapy of primary pneumonias, physiotherapy and tracheostomy care of comatose or ventilated patients, and rapid bronchoscopic clearance of obstructed airways.

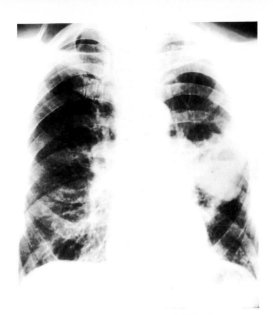

Fig. 133 Post-aspiration lung abscess: fluid level.

38 / Erythema nodosum

Etiology Multiple precipitants including primary tuberculosis, streptococcal disease, intestinal infections (e.g. yersiniosis and campylobacteriosis), sarcoidosis, chronic inflammatory bowel disease and many drugs including combined oral contraceptives.

Incidence Uncommon. Infections are the most common cause in children; acute sarcoid and contraceptive pill in young women.

Pathogenesis A non-infective, non-suppurative localized vasculitis caused by an immunologically mediated' reaction to infective or chemical stimuli, or immunologically based disease.

Clinical features Acutely tender circumscribed erythematous skin nodules, 1–4 cm diameter, usually confined to anterior surface of legs below knees (Figs 134 & 135) but sometimes on extensor surfaces of arms. May appear successively for several weeks but usually settle spontaneously within a few weeks if drug or infection related. May persist or recur in sarcoidosis or auto-immune disease. In acute sarcoidosis erythema nodosum is usually associated with arthritis, hilar adenopathy and fever, and occasionally with phlyctenular conjunctivitis and parotitis.

Diagnosis requires exemplary history taking, search for possible infective or inflammatory causes. Serum ACE, Kveim test and T_{CO} are useful for sarcoidosis. Primary TB must be excluded.

Treatment Removal of etiological factor, e.g. cessation of drugs, eradication of infection or treatment of autoimmune disease. If not contraindicated by etiology (e.g. infections), steroids can have a beneficial effect.

Prevention May require isolation, dependent on causation. Avoidance of previously recognized drug precipitants.

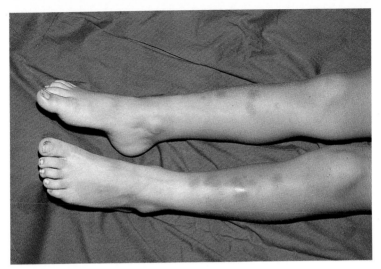

Fig. 134 Early discrete erythema nodosum.

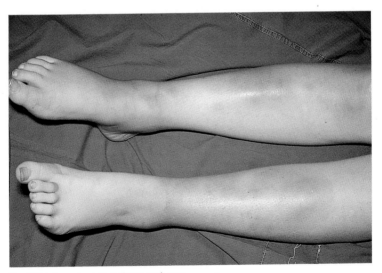

Fig. 135 Late coalescent erythema nodosum.

39 / Stevens–Johnson syndrome

Etiology May complicate therapy with various drugs including sulfonamides and penicillins, and infections caused by herpes simplex, *Mycoplasma pneumoniae* and streptococci.

Incidence Sporadic and uncommon.

Pathogenesis Results from immune hypersensitivity mechanisms of uncertain type which cause vasculitis in the skin, mucous membranes and conjunctivae leading to vesiculobullous lesions.

Clinical features Conjunctival, genital and mucocutaneous lesions of variable severity. Erosive lesions may be found on the lips, buccal mucosa, tongue and genitalia (Figs 136 & 137). Skin lesions are almost invariably present, commonly on the hands and feet, commencing as a multiform eruption subsequently forming vesicles and bullae which may coalesce (Figs 138 & 139). Evolution and regression take place over 2–3 wk and healing may be accompanied by desquamation, skin pigmentation or superficial scarring.

Complications Secondary bacterial skin and oral infection is common. Recurrent herpes simplex infections may precipitate further episodes of Stevens–Johnson syndrome.

Treatment Most cases require symptomatic therapy alone. Secondary skin infections may require treatment with cloxacillin. Alternative therapy is with one of the cephalosporins. Precipitating *M. pneumoniae* infections are treated with erythromycin. Steroids are of unproven benefit.

Prevention Nil presently available. Etiologically-related drugs must be avoided.

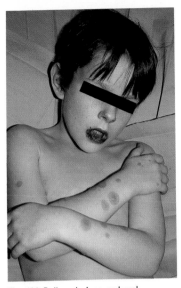

Fig. 136 Bullous lesions and oral ulceration.

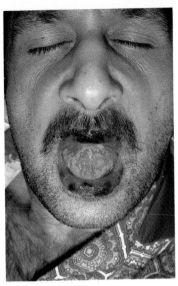

Fig. 137 Ulcers of lips and tongue.

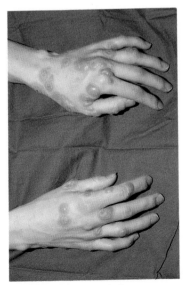

Fig. 138 Vesiculobullous lesions.

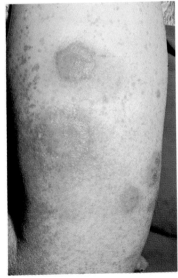

Fig. 139 Bullous lesions (atypical).

40 / **Antibiotic rashes**

Etiology Many antibiotics cause skin rashes, most notably the penicillins, cephalosporins and sulfonamides. Rashes are less commonly caused by erythromycin, chloramphenicol, clindamycin, tetracyclines and quinolones, and only rarely follow the use of aminoglycosides. A maculopapular rash is virtually invariable when patients with glandular fever receive ampicillin (less common with amoxicillin).

Incidence The overall incidence is approximately:
- Penicillins: 2–3% (ampicillin up to 7%).
- Cephalosporins: 1–2% (10% of penicillin-allergic patients also react to cephalosporins).
- Sulfonamides (and co-trimoxazole): 5%.

Pathogenesis Antibiotics may engender immediate hypersensitivity (IgE-mediated) reactions, usually causing urticaria, or delayed reactions both of the serum-sickness (IgG-mediated) type and by other ill-understood mechanisms, including induction of sensitized lymphocytes. The reaction can be due to the parent antibiotic, high molecular weight polymers, or breakdown products.

Clinical features The penicillins, cephalosporins and sulfonamides may all cause urticaria (Fig. 140), morbilliform eruptions (Fig. 141) or erythema multiforme (Fig. 142) and, rarely, Stevens–Johnson syndrome (p. 99).

Complications Drug rashes are usually transient but may be part of a generalized hypersensitivity reaction.

Treatment Early treatment of urticaria with antihistamines or corticosteroids may hasten recovery. Antihistamines are also useful for pruritus associated with morbilliform penicillin/cephalosporin rashes. Treatment is otherwise symptomatic.

Prevention Implicated antibiotics should be avoided in the future.

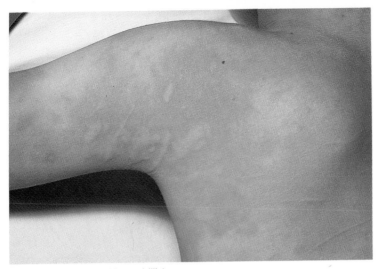

Fig. 140 Urticaria (caused by penicillin).

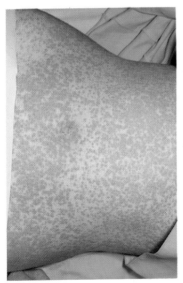

Fig. 141 Morbilliform rash (caused by ampicillin).

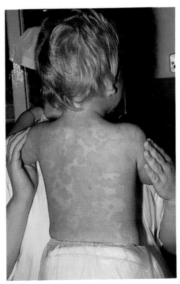

Fig. 142 Erythema multiforme (caused by sulfonamide).

41 / Secondary syphilis

Etiology	*Treponema pallidum*, a spirochete.
Incidence	Worldwide distribution: high incidence in male homosexuals.
Pathogenesis	Sexually transmitted: man is the only host. The local chancre of acquired syphilis starts 9–90 d after sexual contact and is followed 6 wk to several mth later by secondary syphilis. Secondary disease merges into latent endarteritic syphilis in which physical signs are absent but serology, as in secondary syphilis, is positive. Tertiary syphilis causes neurological or cardiovascular disease years later. Secondary syphilis is highly infectious.
Clinical features	Secondary syphilis mimics many skin infections and infestations, including mononucleosis, acute exanthemata, erythema multiforme, condylomata accuminata, alopecia areata and oral or vaginal candidiasis. Macular, maculopapular (Fig. 143), pustular and nodular skin lesions with vesicles last for 1–2 mth. They occur anywhere but mainly on the palms (Fig. 144) and soles. Condylomata lata are non-tender, moist greyish plaques in intertriginous areas, frequently in the perineum. These and mucosal 'snail track' ulcers are highly infectious. Fever, laryngitis, pharyngitis, arthralgia, painless lymphadenopathy and weight loss occur. The diagnosis of secondary syphilis is confirmed by dark-ground examination of exudates for *T. pallidum* and positive serology (TPHA and ELISA for anti-treponemal IgM).
Treatment	Benzathine penicillin G 2.4 million units i.m. weekly × 3 wk or ceftriaxone 250 mg i.m. every other day × 5 doses. Alternatively, erythromycin or tetracycline 500 mg; 6-hourly, for 14 d. The possibility of a Jarisch–Herxheimer reaction may be covered with corticosteroids.

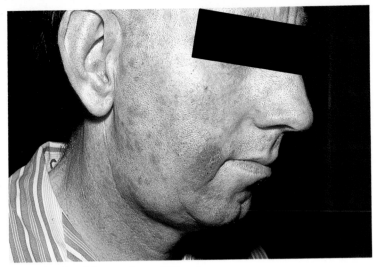

Fig. 143 Papulonodular secondary syphilitic rash.

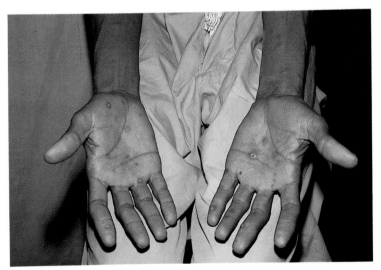

Fig. 144 Palmar lesions in secondary syphilis.

42 / Gonococcemia

Etiology	*Neisseria gonorrhoeae*, a Gram-negative diplococcus.
Incidence	A sporadic complication of genital, anorectal and oropharyngeal gonorrhea.
Pathogenesis	Occurs as a complicating bacteremia with organ involvement in patients with gonorrhea which, in females, may be asymptomatic or, in pharyngeal disease, may be unsuspected.
Clinical features	Initially presents as a pyrexia of unknown origin accompanied by sparse, violaceous macular or vesicular skin lesions (50%) (Figs 145 & 146), or as a pyrexia with organ involvement, most commonly arthritis (80%). Monoarticular septic arthritis usually presents a week or more after onset but polyarticular, hypersensitivity-mediated small joint arthritis may present within a few days. Endocarditis is a later, uncommon complication (5%). Diagnosis is established by blood culture and isolation of *N. gonorrhoeae* from endocervical, vaginal, urethral, anorectal and pharyngeal swabs, or from joint fluid.
	Concomitant syphilis and non-specific genital infection (*Chl. trachomatis*) should be excluded.
Treatment	**For uncomplicated gonococcal urethritis:** ceftriaxone 250 mg i.m. once. Add doxycycline 100 mg p.o. b.i.d. × 7 d or azithromycin 1 g p.o. in a single dose if *Chl. trachomatis* is suspected.
	For penicillin-resistant gonococcemia: cefuroxime, ceftriaxone, cefixime or ciprofloxacin should be given for 7–10 d.
	For complicated gonococcemia (with endocarditis or septic arthritis) at least 4–6 wk treatment is needed.
Prevention	Notifiable: hospitalized cases should be isolated. Routine contact tracing should be undertaken to arrange treatment and prevent secondary disease.

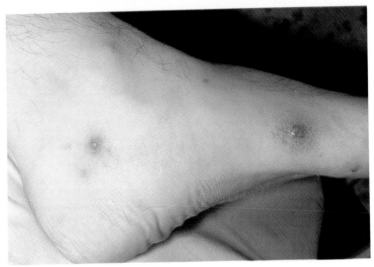

Fig. 145 Violaceous vesicular lesions (iodine self-medication).

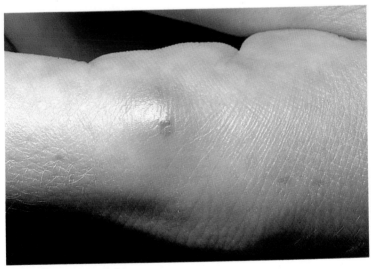

Fig. 146 Papulovesicular lesion.

43 / Acquired immune deficiency syndrome (AIDS)

Etiology   Human immunodeficiency viruses types 1 and 2 (HIV-1/2), RNA retroviruses which attach to CD4 lymphocytes and CNS cells.

Incidence   Worldwide, predominantly caused by HIV-1. Globally more than 10 million individuals have become infected. 1.5 million have developed AIDS and, since the pandemic began, approximately half have already died.

The acquired immune deficiency syndrome (AIDS) was originally recognized as the presence of rare diseases, normally associated with immunodeficiency, e.g. *Pneumocystis carinii* pneumonitis (Fig. 147) or Kaposi's sarcoma (Fig. 148, Fig. 151 (p. 110), & Fig. 153 (p. 112)), in previously healthy homosexual men who were HIV positive. Initially most common as a sexually transmitted infection of homosexuals, AIDS also occurs in drug addicts. HIV infection also spreads heterosexually, notably in Africa (seroprevalence in young sexually active people 30–40%). Such transmission is increasing in the west. Vertical and peri-natal or post-natal infection, e.g. after breast feeding, also occurs.

Pathogenesis   Infection of CNS cells leads to cerebral atrophy and AIDS dementia complex. Continuing virus multiplication in CD4 (T4 helper) lymphocytes causes cell-mediated immunodeficiency. CD4 counts under $200/mm^3$ correlate with onset of symptomatic illness. The incubation period from infection to development of AIDS is often 7–8 yr (less in children). Almost all HIV infections eventually result in AIDS.

Classification   The CDC classification comprises 4 groups. *Group I* is the acute infection, either asymptomatic or resembling glandular fever, after which seroconversion occurs. *Group II* refers to asymptomatic infection, leading either via an intermediate stage (*Group III*) characterized by palpable glands in two or more extra-inguinal sites for >3 months, or directly to *Group IV* (AIDS).

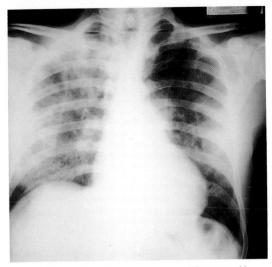

Fig. 147 Chest radiograph: *Pneumocystis carinii* pneumonitis.

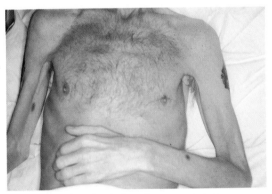

Fig. 148 Cachexia and early Kaposi's sarcoma lesions.

Classification
(contd)

Group IV disease (AIDS) comprises:
- *Group IV A* (AIDS-related complex)—constitutional disease plus either fever, diarrhea for >1 mth or involuntary weight loss of >10% (Fig. 148, p. 108).
- *Group IV B*—CNS disease, myelopathy, neuropathy or dementia.
- *Group IV C1*—infections with *Pneumocystis carinii*, cryptococci, toxoplasma, cryptosporidia, *M. avium-intracellulare*, etc.
- *Group IV C2*—oral hairy leucoplakia, zoster, bacteremic salmonellosis, tuberculosis, etc.
- *Group IV D*—malignancies, KS, cerebral and non-Hodgkin's lymphomas.
- *Group IV E*—chronic lymphoid interstitial pneumonitis (CLIP—normally children) and diseases not otherwise classified.

Clinical features

AIDS commonly presents with PCP: increasing dyspnea reflecting profound hypoxia which worsens dramatically on exercise. Chest X-ray shows diffuse opacification. PCP may also present acutely and pneumothorax can occur. The organism is detected in induced sputum, lavage fluid or tissue from lung biopsy. Children may present with CLIP. Febrile mycobacterial infection is best detected by blood or bone-marrow culture.

Diarrhea may be caused by cryptosporidiosis or salmonellosis but also results from HIV infection, CMV colitis and strongyloidiasis. CMV infections also cause retinitis (Fig. 57, p. 40) and pneumonitis. Esophageal candidosis is also common (Fig. 149). Oral hairy leucoplakia (Fig. 150) is probably viral in origin. Fits, dementia and focal CNS signs may be due to HIV encephalopathy, toxoplasmosis or lymphoma. CSF examination and CT scanning are required. Cryptococcal meningitis presents sub-acutely with fever and headache rather than with meningism.

Male homosexuals often present with Kaposi's sarcoma lesions, typically as purple/brown, painless, non-pruritic areas, flush with the skin or raised strawberry-like skin plaques (Fig. 153, p. 112). Varying initially, they become persistent, enlarge, coalesce, and may bleed. KS can affect internal organs besides producing skin and oral lesions (Fig. 151).

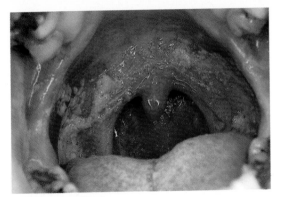

Fig. 149 Oral candidosis.

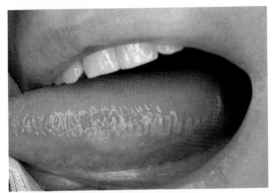

Fig. 150 Oral hairy leukoplakia.

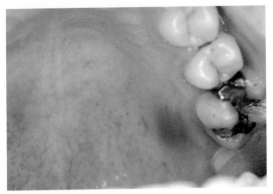

Fig. 151 Kaposi's sarcoma of gums and palate.

In full-blown AIDS, multiple opportunistic infections, tumors and neuropathies commonly co-exist.

Management Counselling, support and education as to avoidance of risk factors are vital. Infected individuals should be regularly monitored both clinically and with full blood and CD4 counts plus estimations of P24 antigen, immunoglobulins and β-2 microglobulin to assess progression of infection. Specific therapy includes:

- *Zidovudine (AZT/Retrovir)*—usually given to symptomatic patients in whom it temporarily increases the CD4 count and may reduce the frequency of opportunistic infections and improve CNS symptoms and HIV retinitis (Fig. 152). Recent studies make its use to delay the onset of AIDS in asymptomatic patients debatable at present.
- *Antitumor* therapy—local radiotherapy, vincristine, vinblastine and bleomycin are useful in KS. Lymphomas respond poorly to cyclophosphamide or standard combination regimens.
- *Antimicrobial chemotherapy*—treated early, PCP responds to high-dose trimethoprim/sulfamethoxazole. Inhaled pentamidine, oral trimethoprim/sulfamethoxazole or dapsone are used to prevent relapse. CMV infections are treated with foscarnet or ganciclovir. Herpes virus infections respond to acyclovir. Superficial mycoses respond to topical nystatin or miconazole; deep infections, e.g. cryptococcosis, to amphotericin B and/or fluconazole. Therapy for cerebral toxoplasmosis and parasitic gut disease, e.g. cryptosporidiosis, is unsatisfactory. Bacterial infections are treated with standard antibiotics.

Prevention Notifiable. No vaccines are currently available. Prevention consists of risk reduction and education. Blood, blood products and donor organs are carefully screened, casual sexual encounters are discouraged and condom use is recommended. Intravenous drug misusers should join withdrawal programs or substitute oral methadone. Sterile needles are supplied by some, but not all, health authorities. Public awareness of HIV infection must be encouraged, in particular the risks of casual unprotected heterosexual intercourse.

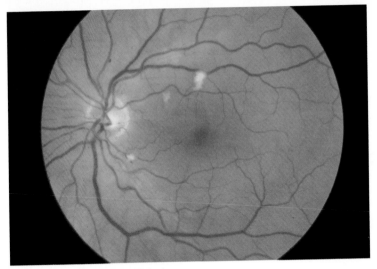

Fig. 152 Retinal exudates in HIV infection.

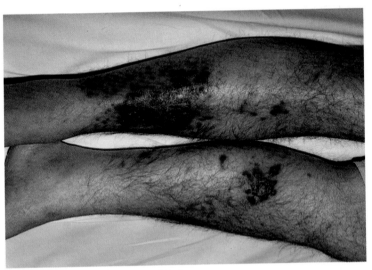

Fig. 153 Extensive Kaposi's sarcoma of the legs.

Index